PATRICIA BRIGHTWELL

Womens Fasting 101

From Beginner to Advanced, Nurturing Youth to Maturity for Enhanced Fat Burning, Radiant Skin, Hormonal Balance, and Boosted Fertility

This book provides an overview and guidance on the possible advantages of fasting. It should not be seen as a substitute for tailored medical advice. Before adopting any health regimen suggested in this book, including fasting practices, it is crucial to seek the counsel of your healthcare provider to ensure it suits your personal health needs. The author and publisher explicitly deny any liability for negative outcomes arising from the implementation of the strategies discussed in this book.

First edition

This book was professionally typeset on Reedsy.
Find out more at reedsy.com

"Change starts now it's an action we take today not tomorrow. Results are from actions we took yesterday."

Patricia Brightwell

Contents

Introduction

After the birth of my third child, finding my way back to my pre-pregnancy weight felt like an impossible challenge. Like many women, I found myself navigating through a labyrinth of diets, from ultra-restrictive caloric regimes to vegetarian and even vegan pathways. Despite squeezing in exercise whenever possible, weeks turned into months with minimal progress. The scale barely budged, and the energy I had invested seemed to vanish into thin air, leaving me exhausted and disheartened. It was only when I stumbled upon the concept of fasting that the tide began to turn. Within about a week of adopting a fasting routine, I shed 5 pounds – a feat I hadn't achieved in months. This breakthrough was about weight loss and reclaiming control over my health and life.

This book is crafted to guide women, irrespective of their age or life stage, through the transformative journey of fasting. From the novice embarking on her first fast to the seasoned faster seeking to refine her approach, this guide addresses the unique considerations women face - hormonal fluctuations, menstrual cycles, and emotional health, all while targeting weight loss and vitality restoration.

Directed towards women seeking a sustainable and effective avenue to shed pounds, rejuvenate health, and recapture youth, this book embraces readers from diverse backgrounds and health statuses. It's structured to unfold the mysteries of fasting, starting with foundational knowledge, progressing to customizing fasting plans, exploring advanced techniques, and integrating fasting into a lifestyle poised for longevity. This book is not a one-size-fits-all fasting manual; it's a deep dive into fasting with a woman's physiological and hormonal blueprint in mind.

Empowerment through knowledge is a central theme of our journey together. By equipping you with the tools and insights to navigate fasting effectively, this book aims to transform the way you approach health and wellness. Peppered with personal success stories, including my own, these narratives serve as beacons of hope and evidence of what's possible when we align our lifestyle with our body's natural rhythms.

Fasting can seem intimidating, perhaps even controversial, to some. This book is prepared to dismantle those doubts, armed with evidence-based benefits tailored to women's needs. As we embark on this journey together, please keep an open mind and steadfastly commit yourself.

Fasting is more than a dietary choice; it's a pathway to rediscovery. It's about unearthing the strength to transform your body and your entire outlook on health and life. Let this be the moment you step into a future brimming with health, vitality, and confidence. Welcome to your fasting journey—a journey to the best version of yourself.

Chapter 1: The Science of Fasting for Women

What is fasting?

F asting is voluntarily abstaining from food and, sometimes, fluids for a predetermined period. This process triggers a series of metabolic and cellular responses within the body due to the absence of incoming energy sources from food. Initially, the body utilizes glucose stored in the liver as glycogen for energy. Once these stores are depleted, typically after about 12 to 36 hours, the body transitions to breaking down fat for energy, known as ketosis. This shift not only aids in weight loss and improves metabolic health but also enhances insulin sensitivity, reducing the risk of type 2 diabetes.

Autophagy is a woman's secret weapon for youth.

A significant biological process induced during fasting is autophagy, the body's mechanism of cleaning out damaged cells and regenerating new ones. This process, which gets activated during prolonged periods of fasting, is crucial for cellular repair and maintenance. It helps remove protein aggregates and dysfunctional organelles, reducing inflammation and improving cellular function. Autophagy is linked to increased longevity, improved brain function, and a reduced risk of diseases, including neurodegenerative disorders and cancer. Fasting can offer numerous health benefits through these complex biological mechanisms, from improved metabolic health to enhanced cellular renewal and disease prevention.

Aging benefits of autophagy

Autophagy emerges as a beacon of hope in the quest for longevity and the elixir of youth, particularly for women navigating the intricacies of aging. This self-cleansing mechanism, where our cells diligently recycle their worn-out parts, holds the secret to slowing the aging process and potentially reversing it. Autophagy offers a promising pathway to preserving vitality and youthfulness for women whose bodies undergo many hormonal changes through the years.

As we age, accumulating damaged cells and proteins can accelerate physical health and appearance decline. Autophagy, however, acts as a natural detoxification process, clearing away the cellular debris that contributes to aging. This not only aids in reducing inflammation, a key player in the aging narrative but also enhances cellular function, ensuring our organs and skin retain their youthful vigor longer.

For women, the benefits of stimulating autophagy extend beyond mere aesthetics. It bolsters immune function, reduces the risk of age-related diseases, and supports hormonal balance, addressing issues from menstrual irregularities to menopausal transitions gracefully. Engaging in practices that promote autophagy, such as fasting, exercising, and consuming autophagy-inducing nutrients, can be transformative. It empowers women to take control of their aging process, offering a pathway to a more extended life filled with vitality and radiance.

Impact on skin and beauty

In the realm of beauty and skin health, the impact of autophagy stands out as a testament to nature's rejuvenating process. This cellular renewal mechanism, when activated, offers profound benefits for the skin, particularly for women who often turn to countless creams and treatments in pursuit of youthful radiance. Autophagy delicately peels away the layers of accumulated damage, revealing a canvas of vitality and reduced signs of aging.

Imagine the skin as a garden that thrives on meticulous care—autophagy is akin to the gardener meticulously removing dead foliage to make way for new growth. This natural cleansing process targets the foundation of skin health by eliminating damaged proteins and organelles, thus preventing the dullness, wrinkles, and sagging that often accompany aging. The result is a visible enhancement in skin texture and firmness, a reduction in fine lines and age spots, and an overall luminous complexion.

For women, the allure of autophagy lies in its ability to harmonize with the body's innate rhythms, supporting skin elasticity and hydration without invasive treatments. It's a holistic approach to beauty that aligns with the principles of self-care and wellness, offering a sustainable path to maintaining a youthful glow. By embracing lifestyle choices that stimulate autophagy, women can unlock the secret to enduring beauty that flourishes from within and withstands the test of time.

Optimizing Autophagy

For women seeking to harness the transformative power of autophagy, the journey to optimal health and vitality is beautifully interwoven with intentional lifestyle choices and fasting methods. Fasting, in various forms, catalyzes autophagy, inviting the body to initiate its internal cleansing and renewal process. This ancient practice, ranging from intermittent to extended fasting periods, allows women to align with their body's natural rhythms, promoting cellular repair and rejuvenation.

Intermittent fasting, with its flexible approach, fits seamlessly into the ebb and flow of a woman's life, offering a gentle yet effective way to stimulate autophagy without overwhelming the body. For those seeking more profound cellular renewal, periodic extended fasts serve as a deep reset, amplifying the autophagic process and its myriad benefits. We will go over the various methods throughout the book.

Complementing these fasting strategies with lifestyle choices that nurture the body and soul elevates the autophagy experience. A diet rich in phytonutrients, regular physical activity, and mindfulness practices like yoga and meditation support autophagy and cultivate a sense of holistic well-being. By embracing these practices, women can unlock a symphony of health benefits, weaving the art of fasting with the science of longevity to create a tapestry of vibrant health and timeless beauty.

Why fasting is different for women HORMONES

The role of hormones in fasting

In the intricate dance of fasting and health, hormones play a pivotal role, especially for women, whose bodies exhibit a heightened sensitivity to fluctuations in energy intake. This delicate balance influences vital players in our endocrine orchestra—insulin, ghrelin, and leptin—each responding uniquely to the rhythms of fasting and feeding.

Insulin, the conductor of glucose metabolism, sees its levels modulate with fasting, enhancing insulin sensitivity. This adjustment is particularly beneficial for women, supporting balanced blood sugar levels and reducing the risk of metabolic conditions. Ghrelin, known as the hunger hormone, sings its siren song, adjusting its levels to signal satiety and hunger. Fasting tempers ghrelin's call, fine-tuning our body's hunger cues, and aiding in mindful food consumption.

Leptin, the hormone responsible for signaling fullness, is also crucial. As women begin fasting, leptin sensitivity can improve, fostering a healthier relationship with food and satiety. This symphony of hormonal adjustments underlines the unique experience women have with fasting. By understanding and respecting these hormonal sensitivities, women can tailor fasting practices to harness these benefits fully, ensuring that the journey toward health and vitality is compelling and harmonious.

Fasting Can Increase Fertility and Conception

Fasting casts a profound influence on women's reproductive health, weaving its effects through the delicate tapestry of reproductive hormones. This ancient practice is critical to unlocking a harmonious balance within, potentially enhancing menstrual cycle regularity and fostering fertility. The interplay between fasting and reproductive health illuminates the body's ability to adapt and thrive under varying energy intake conditions.

As women embark on fasting, they may discover a gentle recalibration of their menstrual cycles. This phenomenon is rooted in the body's response to changes in nutritional intake, which affects the hormonal balance crucial for reproductive functions. Fasting can modulate the levels of hormones such as estrogen and progesterone, pivotal in the menstrual cycle's orchestration, promoting regularity and easing symptoms associated with hormonal imbalances.

Furthermore, the impact of fasting on fertility is a subject of growing interest and optimism. By improving insulin sensitivity and reducing inflammation, fasting may enhance ovarian function and egg quality, offering a beacon of hope for those navigating fertility challenges. When embraced thoughtfully and aligned with one's body signals, this holistic approach can support the intricate dance of reproductive health, paving a path toward enhanced well-being and the potential for conception.

Adrenal and Thyroid Health

Embarking on the path of fasting introduces women to a nuanced dialogue between their body's energy management systems and their wellness aspirations, particularly concerning adrenal and thyroid health. These glands, though small, are mighty conductors of our metabolic harmony and energy symphony. Fasting, with its rhythmic ebb and flow of energy intake, plays a fascinating role in this delicate balance, offering insights into the body's resilience and adaptability.

Fasting is a double-edged sword for the adrenal glands that manage stress through cortisol secretion. Thoughtfully integrated fasting regimens can encourage a beneficial reset, reducing stress on the adrenal system and promoting a more balanced cortisol response. This careful modulation supports sustained energy levels and a serene mental state, essential for thriving in today's fast-paced world.

The thyroid gland, the maestro of metabolism, also responds to the subtle cues of fasting. By influencing insulin sensitivity and hormonal balance, fasting may foster an environment conducive to optimal thyroid function.

This can translate to a more vibrant metabolism, enhancing energy levels and facilitating weight management. However, the key lies in mindful practice and listening deeply to one's body, ensuring that fasting is a gentle nudge toward health rather than an overwhelming challenge. In this way, women can harness fasting's potential to nurture their adrenal and thyroid health, stepping gracefully into a state of empowered well-being.

Customizing Fasting plans to meet your hormone needs

In fasting, the notion that one size fits all dissolves like mist under the morning sun, especially for women whose bodies narrate stories of cyclical change and hormonal ebb and flow. Customizing fasting plans becomes not just a consideration but a necessity, a gentle acknowledgment of the unique rhythms that govern female physiology. This tailored approach ensures that fasting becomes a harmonious ally to health rather than a disruptive force.

Recognizing the nuances of hormonal fluctuations across the menstrual cycle, menopause, and various life stages empowers women to align their fasting practices with their body's intrinsic needs. A customized fasting plan can accommodate heightened sensitivity or energy demands, adjusting fasting durations and intensity to support rather than challenge hormonal balance. This mindful synchronization offers a path to enhance well-being, optimize health outcomes, and embrace fasting as a sustainable practice.

Tailoring fasting plans allows for a compassionate and informed engagement with one's health, honoring the body's signals and seasons. It paves the way for a deeper connection with one's wellness journey, transforming fasting into a nurturing space of self-care and discovery. For women, customizing fasting plans becomes an act of empowerment, enabling them to navigate their health landscapes with grace, understanding, and respect for their body's profound wisdom.

Debunking Fasting Myths: What Every Woman Needs to Know

Myth: Fasting is Unsafe for Women

In the tapestry of health and wellness, fasting emerges as a practice shrouded in myths, particularly the pervasive misconception that it poses inherent dangers to women. While rooted in concerns for well-being, this narrative often overlooks the burgeoning body of scientific evidence illuminating fasting's benefits. Women must navigate these waters armed with knowledge, discerning myth from truth, to embrace practices that enrich their health.

The myth that fasting is unsafe for women stems from fears of nutritional deficiencies and hormonal imbalances. However, when approached with mindfulness and tailored to individual health needs, fasting is a potent ally, enhancing metabolic flexibility, supporting hormonal health, and promoting autophagy. Scientific studies underscore fasting's role in improving insulin sensitivity, reducing inflammation, and even bolstering cognitive function, offering a counter-narrative to the myth of danger.

Understanding that women's bodies are uniquely responsive to changes in energy intake, the key lies in customizing fasting protocols. Intermittent fasting, cyclic fasting, and other adaptable approaches allow for the integration of fasting into women's lives in a way that supports rather than undermines health. By debunking the myth of fasting's inherent danger, women can confidently explore fasting as a transformative tool, unlocking pathways to vitality, longevity, and empowered well-being.

Myth: Fasting Leads to Eating Disorders

The journey of fasting, while transformative, is often clouded by the myth that it paves the way to eating disorders. This misconception arises from a genuine concern for mental and physical health, yet it simplifies the nuanced relationship between fasting and eating behaviors. Navigating this conversation with empathy, understanding, and evidence is essential, highlighting the distinction between mindful fasting and disordered eating patterns.

Fasting, when embraced as a conscious, health-oriented practice, encourages a deeper connection with the body's hunger and fullness cues, fostering an environment of mindful eating. This intentionality stands in stark contrast to the compulsive behaviors characteristic of eating disorders. Rather than precipitating disordered eating, a carefully curated approach to fasting can empower individuals to reclaim agency over their dietary choices, enhancing their relationship with food through intentional eating and fasting periods.

The key to harnessing the benefits of fasting while safeguarding against potential risks lies in its application with awareness and respect for one's body signals. Engaging in fasting as part of a holistic approach to health, underpinned by education and guidance from healthcare professionals, can mitigate concerns related to eating disorders. By debunking this myth, we illuminate fasting's potential as a pathway to physical rejuvenation and a balanced and mindful approach to eating.

Myth: Fasting Causes Muscle Loss

The myth that fasting inevitably leads to muscle loss casts a shadow over its many benefits, especially for women seeking strength and vitality. This misconception overlooks the body's remarkable adaptability and the strategic approaches that can preserve and even enhance muscle mass during periods of fasting.

Fasting initiates a symphony of metabolic adjustments, not a reckless dismantling of muscle tissue, as the myth suggests. In its wisdom, the body prefers to burn stored fat for energy before it turns to muscle, especially when fasting is paired with strategic nutrition and exercise. Incorporating periods of protein-rich eating and resistance training into the fasting routine ensures the maintenance of muscle mass. Amino acids from protein support muscle repair and growth, while strength training stimulates muscles, signaling the body to preserve muscle tissue even in a fasted state.

Thus, Women can navigate fasting confidently, knowing that muscle mass can be protected and even augmented through mindful dietary choices and consistent physical activity. By debunking the myth of inevitable muscle loss, fasting is revealed not as a threat but as an ally to women seeking a balanced approach to health, empowering them to achieve their wellness goals without sacrificing strength.

Myth: All Fasting Plans Are the Same

The myth that all fasting plans are cast from the same mold fails to capture the rich tapestry of approaches and their distinct impacts on health and well-being. This blanket assumption overlooks the nuanced nature of fasting, where the diversity of methods—from intermittent fasting to extended fasts—caters to each individual's unique rhythms and needs. As each body is a universe unto itself, each fasting plan offers a constellation of benefits tailored to the voyager's journey.

Intermittent fasting, with its cycles of eating and fasting, may suit those seeking flexibility and balance, while time-restricted feeding, focusing on the timing of meals, appeals to those aiming to align their eating patterns with their circadian rhythms. Extended fasting, venturing into more prolonged periods of fasting, offers profound metabolic reset opportunities. Each method activates the body's healing mechanisms, influencing everything from weight loss and energy levels to cellular repair and mental clarity.

Emphasizing personalization is critical; what works as a transformative practice for one may not suit another. Understanding one's health status, goals, and lifestyle allows for the customization of fasting plans, ensuring they nourish and empower rather than deplete. By dispelling the myth of uniformity, we open the door to a world of fasting practices rich in variety and potential, inviting each individual to discover the fasting path that resonates most profoundly with their unique journey to health and vitality.

Chapter 2: Fasting Safely - Starting Your Journey

Identifying Your Fasting Type: Personalized Strategies

E mbarking on the fasting journey for women is akin to navigating a lush, diverse forest; the selected route must resonate with her unique landscape of health goals, lifestyle, and personal nuances. This is not just about choosing a fasting method; it's about embracing a discovery process that honors a woman's intricate physiological rhythms, aspirations, and daily commitments. Such a personalized approach ensures that fasting becomes a practice and a sustainable part of her lifestyle, enriching her journey toward health and vitality.

For women taking their first steps into fasting, intermittent fasting offers a welcoming gateway. Its flexible cycles of eating and fasting adapt seamlessly to the rhythm of daily life, supporting goals from weight management to improved metabolic health, all while fostering a mindful connection with food.

Time-restricted feeding, which narrows the eating window to daylight hours, is particularly suited to women looking to align their eating patterns with their circadian rhythms. This approach promises enhanced energy levels throughout the day and improved sleep quality, which is crucial for a woman's holistic well-being.

Extended fasting, which stretches beyond 24 hours, might appeal to those seeking a profound metabolic reset and the deep cellular renewal of autophagy. Though more intense, this method can be transformative, especially when approached with mindfulness of one's physical readiness and lifestyle needs.

Identifying a fasting type involves self-reflection. If you have health concerns, consult a healthcare provider and start with a method that feels intuitive and manageable. A tailored strategy amplifies the benefits of fasting, weaving it into the fabric of your life in a way that nurtures and empowers, reflecting the unique journey each woman undertakes toward her health and vitality.

Now, let's take a quick look at the types of fasting: intermittent or time-restrictive eating and traditional fasting or extended fasting. Intermittent fasting consists of eating at different times around or within 24 hours. These methods focus mainly on the time window of when you will eat. Traditional and extended fasting is more about complete abstinence from food and sometimes liquids for a continuous period, usually at least 24 hrs. Women aiming for deeper cellular repair, autophagy, significant weight loss, and enhanced insulin sensitivity will enjoy the benefits of these longer fasts. Unlike intermittent fasting, traditional or extended fasting doesn't focus on when you eat but the fasting period itself.

Transitioning from burning glucose (sugar) for energy to burning fat can vary significantly among individuals, depending on various factors, including their metabolic rate, diet, and physical activity levels. However, a commonly referenced point at which the body shifts towards burning fat for energy is after glycogen stores in the liver are depleted, typically after about 12 to 36 hours of fasting. But through intermittent fasting, you can achieve depletion of glycogen stores slower over time, still leading to ketosis. Although a longer fast can get you into ketosis faster. Some like to transition smoothly, while some want results now and are willing to be uncomfortable for a day; eventually, it will become easier. Once you experience the benefits, you will look forward to your fasting days and the benefits that come with them.

Intermittent Fasting Methods

Intermittent Fasting has become a popular approach to wellness, with various methods offering unique benefits tailored to individual health goals, lifestyles, and preferences. Understanding these different fasting types can empower women to choose the most suitable method that meets their needs. Here's an overview of the most common fasting methods:

16/8 Method:

- Fasting for 16 hours and eating within an 8-hour window each day.
- Suitable for Women seeking a sustainable and flexible approach to weight loss, improved insulin sensitivity, and enhanced mental clarity.
- It is ideal for those who prefer a consistent routine and can easily skip breakfast or dinner.
- The easiest method to start with
- Start here if you have never fasted before
- One Meal A Day (OMAD):
- Consuming all daily calories in a single meal, typically within a 1-hour eating window.
- Suitable for Women looking for significant weight loss results and more profound metabolic health improvements.
- Best for individuals with a flexible schedule that allows for a substantial meal once a day, ensuring nutrient-dense food choices.

5:2 Method:

- I generally eat five days a week and reduce calorie intake to about 500-600 calories on two non-consecutive days.
- Suitable for Women aiming for weight loss without drastic daily restrictions and those interested in longevity and reduced inflammation.
- It fits well with busy lifestyles, offering flexibility on reduced-calorie days to plan around social or work commitments.

Alternate-Day Fasting (ADF):

- Alternating between days of normal eating and days of no or minimal calorie intake (about 500 calories).
- Suitable for Women seeking significant weight loss, improved cardiovascular health, and autophagy benefits.
- Requires a high degree of flexibility and resilience, suitable for those who can handle significant calorie variation.

Eat-Stop-Eat:

- Involves 24-hour fasts once or twice a week, starting from one meal to the same meal the next day.
- Suitable for Women interested in weight loss, detoxification, and discipline in eating habits.
- Ideal for those who can commit to full-day fasts without impacting energy levels for daily activities.

Each fasting method offers different pathways to achieving health and wellness goals. Women considering fasting should consider their nutritional needs, daily routines, and how their bodies respond to periods of fasting, especially concerning menstrual cycles and hormonal changes. Consulting with a healthcare provider before a fasting regimen can provide additional guidance tailored to individual health conditions and goals.

If you have experience with fasting, you can choose any method or start with the length of time you are comfortable with. Starting with the shortest is advised if you are a beginner or it's your first time. As you are successful, you can increase the time window. This will allow your body to acclimate to fasting. Abrupt changes or suddenly stopping all calorie intake can be hard on your body and very uncomfortable. Sudden drastic changes are not recommended. Building your fasting regimen over time will help you be successful.

Fasting more than 24 hrs

Extended Fasting:

- Refers to fasting periods lasting longer than 24 hours, often 24 to 72 hours, without consuming any calories.
- Suitable for women aiming for deeper cellular repair, autophagy, significant weight loss, and enhanced insulin sensitivity.
- Best for individuals with experience in shorter fasts, looking to deepen their fasting practice, and can commit to more extended periods without food.

Assessing Your Health Status

Before embarking on the transformative journey of fasting, women must lay the foundation of this voyage by assessing their current health status. This initial step is not merely a precaution but a beacon guiding the way toward a fasting method that harmonizes with the body's unique needs and rhythms. Evaluating one's health involves a thoughtful reflection on existing medical conditions, nutritional requirements, and overall well-being, ensuring that the chosen fasting path nurtures rather than challenges the body.

For women, this assessment is particularly crucial due to the intricate dance of hormonal fluctuations and the potential impact on reproductive health, bone density, and mental well-being. Conditions such as diabetes, hypothyroidism, or a history of eating disorders require careful consideration and possibly adaptation of fasting practices to accommodate these concerns. Consulting with a healthcare provider can offer invaluable insights, tailoring fasting strategies to support health goals while safeguarding against adverse effects.

This personalized approach empowers women to embrace fasting as a tool for empowerment, enhancing their health journey with mindfulness and care. By aligning fasting practices with their health status, women can unlock the full benefits of fasting, from revitalized energy and improved metabolic health to a profound sense of well-being while navigating the journey with wisdom and grace.

Lifestyle Compatibility

Selecting a fasting method that resonates with the rhythm of your life is akin to choosing a dance partner; it requires harmony, understanding, and a mutual flow. For women, integrating fasting into their daily lives demands a thoughtful consideration of lifestyle compatibility. This ensures that the practice enhances, rather than disrupts, their daily routine, work schedule, and personal preferences. It's about weaving fasting into the fabric of your life in a way that feels natural and supportive.

Begin by reflecting on the contours of your typical day: the demands of your job, family responsibilities, social engagements, and personal downtime. Consider how different fasting schedules might complement these elements. For instance, if mornings are hectic, a method that skips breakfast, like the 16/8 intermittent fasting, might seamlessly fit into your lifestyle. Alternatively, a fasting plan accommodating evening meals would be more appropriate if you cherish dinner with your family as a daily ritual.

Moreover, ponder your preferences and how they align with various fasting methods. If you value flexibility and minimal disruption, intermittent fasting or time-restricted eating might be your allies. For those drawn to more profound, more reflective fasting experiences, extended fasts or the 5:2 method may offer the deep engagement you seek.

Ultimately, the fasting type you choose should feel like a supportive companion, enhancing your health and well-being while respecting the unique tapestry of your life. This thoughtful alignment between fasting and lifestyle ensures sustainability and enriches your journey toward holistic health.

Fasting Through the Ages: Adapting Your Approach as You Mature

Fasting in Your 20s and 30s

Fasting in your 20s and 30s presents an exquisite opportunity to nurture your body, supporting hormonal balance, fertility, and metabolic health during these pivotal decades. As women navigate the complexities of early adulthood, careers, and perhaps the beginning of their journey into motherhood, fasting can be a graceful ally, offering benefits that resonate deeply with their evolving needs.

Tailoring fasting strategies during these years involves a mindful approach that respects the body's hormonal ebb and flow. Intermittent fasting, particularly the 16/8 method, can seamlessly integrate into the dynamic lifestyles of women in their 20s and 30s, supporting insulin sensitivity and aiding in weight management without compromising energy levels or nutritional needs.

For those focused on fertility, adopting a gentle fasting regimen can support reproductive health, enhancing hormonal harmony and potentially improving outcomes for those trying to conceive. It's crucial to ensure that fasting practices are moderated to avoid undue stress on the body, aligning with cycles of rest and nourishment that foster a fertile ground for conception.

Incorporating nutrient-dense foods during eating windows, focusing on whole foods rich in vitamins, minerals, and antioxidants, further amplifies fasting's benefits, ensuring that metabolic health is bolstered while supporting the body's intricate hormonal dance.

As women in their 20s and 30s embrace fasting, doing so with awareness, flexibility, and a deep respect for their body's signals ensures that this practice becomes a powerful tool in their wellness arsenal, supporting their journey towards optimal health, vitality, and fertility.

Navigating Fasting in Your 40s and 50s

Navigating the transition through your 40s and 50s, women encounter the profound shifts of perimenopause and menopause, stages marked by significant hormonal changes that can influence weight, mood, and overall health. During these decades, fasting emerges not just as a dietary choice but a strategic companion, offering a means to gracefully manage these transitions, focusing on weight management and hormonal health.

Adjusting fasting approaches to accommodate the nuances of peri-menopause and menopause involves a nuanced understanding of one's body and its changing needs. Intermittent fasting, particularly in the form of a gentle 14/10 or 16/8 schedule, can be particularly beneficial, helping to stabilize insulin levels and mitigate the typical weight gain associated with these life stages. This form of fasting supports metabolic flexibility, which is crucial as the body's metabolism naturally slows with age.

Moreover, fasting during these years can aid in addressing the hormonal fluctuations of perimenopause and menopause, reducing inflammation, and improving cellular function. However, it's essential to approach fasting with balance and mindfulness, ensuring adequate nutrient intake during eating windows to support bone health, maintain muscle mass, and nurture overall well-being.

Women in their 40s and 50s might find that integrating fasting into their lifestyle, with adjustments for intensity and duration, offers a pathway to manage weight and hormonal health and embrace these years with vitality and grace. By listening to their bodies and consulting with healthcare profes-sionals, they can tailor fasting practices to thrive during this transformative period.

Fasting Beyond 60

Fasting beyond age 60 unfolds as a journey of discovery, an opportunity to gracefully embrace longevity, vitality, and well-being. For women navigating post-menopausal years, fasting offers a powerful tool to manage the physio-logical changes accompanying aging and as a proactive strategy for cognitive health and disease prevention.

Implementing fasting safely in these later years requires a thoughtful approach, considering the body's nutritional needs and capacity for resilience.

Intermittent fasting, with its adaptable frameworks like the 16/8 or even a more gentle 12/12 schedule, can integrate seamlessly into daily life, supporting metabolic health and aiding in managing body weight, which often becomes a challenge with advancing age.

Beyond weight management, fasting in later years promises to enhance cognitive function and offer protective benefits against age-related diseases. The process of autophagy, stimulated by fasting, plays a crucial role in cellular cleanup and renewal, potentially lowering the risk of developing neurodegenerative diseases and fostering a sense of mental clarity and vitality.

Moreover, fasting can contribute to a more balanced hormonal landscape even after menopause, helping mitigate some lingering effects of hormonal changes on mood, energy levels, and overall well-being.

For women over 60, integrating fasting into their lifestyle with an emphasis on moderation, mindful nutrition, and perhaps consultation with healthcare professionals can pave the way for a vibrant, healthful, and fulfilling journey into later life, marked by embracing longevity and a proactive stance against aging.

Life Stage Adjustments

As women journey through the tapestry of life, from the bloom of youth into the wisdom of age, their bodies and needs evolve profoundly. Each life stage—be it the fertile years, the transformative time of pregnancy and motherhood, the shifting sands of perimenopause and menopause, or the serene grace of the post-menopausal years—brings unique challenges and opportunities for growth. Recognizing the importance of modifying fasting techniques to align with these transitions is pivotal in supporting a woman's overall well-being, ensuring that her approach to fasting nurtures her body at every turn.

Adapting fasting practices to accommodate the body's changing hormonal landscape is not just wise; it's an act of self-care that honors the body's innate wisdom and capacity for adaptation. Fasting can be tailored to support hormonal balance and fertility in the reproductive years. As women enter perimenopause and menopause, adjusting fasting schedules can help manage weight, mood fluctuations, and other symptoms associated with hormonal changes. Beyond menopause, fasting continues to offer benefits for longevity, cognitive health, and disease prevention, with adjustments ensuring these practices remain nurturing and beneficial.

Embracing life-stage adjustments in fasting practices empowers women to listen deeply to their bodies, responding with kindness and flexibility. It's a journey of attunement, allowing fasting to be a supportive companion that evolves alongside them, enhancing their health, vitality, and well-being through every chapter of life.

Experimentation and Adjustment

Embarking on a fasting journey invites women to adopt an experimental mindset, transforming the quest for health and vitality into a personal exploration of what truly resonates with their bodies and lives. This approach is not about adhering rigidly to prescribed methods but about encouraging curiosity, flexibility, and a willingness to adjust. It's about crafting a fasting routine that is effective and joyfully sustainable.

Experimentation in fasting allows women to tune into their body's signals, discovering which fasting schedules enhance their energy, which foods nourish their bodies during eating windows, and how their fasting practices can flexibly adapt to life's ever-changing rhythms. This process of trial and adjustment acknowledges that what works marvelously at one life stage or season may need reevaluation and modification as circumstances evolve.

By engaging with fasting in this dynamic way, women empower themselves to balance discipline, gentleness, structure, and fluidity. They learn to navigate the fasting landscape with intuition and insight, making informed adjustments that honor their health goals, lifestyle demands, and personal preferences.

Encouraging an experimental mindset towards fasting fosters a deep, personal connection to wellness, where each woman becomes the expert on her body and journey. With curiosity and adaptable strategies, this path leads to physical health and a profound sense of self-awareness and fulfillment.

The First Fast: Setting Yourself Up for Success

Setting Realistic Goals

Embarking on your first fast is a step into a realm of empowerment, a journey that begins with the foundation of setting realistic goals. This initial foray into fasting is not just about the physical act of refraining from eating for a set period; it's about nurturing confidence, building momentum, and crafting a positive relationship with this transformative practice. For women, especially, aligning the first fasting experience with achievable, gentle goals paves the way for a journey marked by self-discovery and wellness.

Starting with attainable fasting goals—such as a shorter fasting window in the 12/12 or 16/8 method—allows for a gradual introduction to the practice, ensuring that the body and mind can adapt without feeling overwhelmed. This approach fosters a sense of Achievement and encourages the cultivation of patience and kindness towards oneself, essential qualities for sustaining a fasting practice over time.

Moreover, setting realistic goals for your first fast invites a reflective process, encouraging women to consider their motivations, health status, and lifestyle. It's about creating a fasting experience that feels supportive, not punitive, allowing for adjustments and learning.

As you stand at the threshold of your fasting journey, remember that success lies not in the extremes but in the sustainable steps forward. By setting achievable goals for your first fast, you're not just preparing for a period of abstention but laying the groundwork for a lifelong path to health and vitality that honors your body's rhythms and personal growth.

Preparation is vital

As you approach the threshold of your first fast, preparation emerges as the cornerstone of success, a harmonious blend of mental readiness and physical groundwork. This preparatory phase is not merely logistical; it's a nurturing process that aligns your body and spirit with the forthcoming journey. For women, who often juggle myriad responsibilities and roles, this careful orchestration ensures that the fasting experience becomes a source of strength and rejuvenation rather than a challenge to endure.

Mental Preparation:

Embarking on a fast requires a mindset of resilience and openness. Cultivate a supportive internal dialogue, reminding yourself of the reasons behind your fasting decision—be it for health, self-care, or exploration. Visualizing your fasting days and anticipating how you might handle potential challenges can fortify your resolve and help you approach fasting confidently and calmly.

Physical Preparation:

Make gentle dietary adjustments in the days leading up to your fast. Gradually reduce your sugars, processed foods, and caffeine intake while increasing hydration and focusing on whole, nutrient-dense foods. This shift eases the transition into fasting and minimizes potential discomforts like headaches or cravings.

Scheduling:

Choose a fasting window that harmonizes with your daily routine, ensuring it complements your natural rhythms and commitments. Planning your fasting days during less demanding periods can help maintain your energy levels and focus, making the experience more manageable and enjoyable.

By laying the groundwork with thoughtful preparation, you're not just setting the stage for your first fast but nurturing a foundation of self-care that will support you throughout this transformative journey. This mental and physical preparation is a profound act of self-love, setting you up for success and a deeper connection with your body's innate wisdom.

Managing Expectations

As you embark on the transformative path of fasting, managing expectations becomes a vital compass, guiding you through the initial challenges with grace and resilience. It's essential to acknowledge that these early hurdles are not just obstacles but stepping stones on your journey to wellness. For women, who often balance a delicate interplay of responsibilities, understanding and accepting these challenges can empower them to stay motivated and committed to their fasting journey.

The initial foray into fasting may bring moments of hunger, fluctuations in energy, and emotional ups and downs. These experiences, though perhaps uncomfortable, are expected and indicative of your body's adaptation to a new rhythm of nourishment. Embrace these signs not as signs of failure but as markers of transformation, your body's natural response to change.

Staying motivated through these early hurdles requires a blend of self-compassion and perseverance. Celebrate the small victories—a successfully completed fasting day, the newfound clarity of mind, or even the simple act of listening deeply to your body's needs. Find support in communities of like-minded individuals, where shared experiences and encouragement can bolster your resolve.

Remember, the fasting journey is as much about inner discovery as about health. By managing your expectations and embracing the challenges with an open heart, you pave the way for an enriching journey. This journey is not just about the destination but about growing stronger, wiser, and more attuned to your body's needs with each step.

Support systems

Navigating the fasting journey is akin to embarking on a voyage of self-discovery and transformation. Along this path, the power of community—whether found online or in person—becomes an invaluable source of support, inspiration, and camaraderie. For women, tapping into these support systems can significantly enhance the fasting experience, providing a wellspring of motivation, shared wisdom, and encouragement.

Leveraging community support involves actively seeking out forums, social media groups, or local meetups where experiences, challenges, and successes related to fasting are openly shared. In these spaces, women can find not only practical advice and tips but also emotional support from others who understand the intricacies of the journey. This sense of belonging and connection can be incredibly empowering during moments of doubt or when navigating the initial hurdles of fasting.

Engaging with a fasting community encourages accountability, crucial in maintaining a commitment to fasting goals. Sharing your journey, in turn, contributes to the collective knowledge and support network, fostering a reciprocal relationship of giving and receiving support.

Moreover, these communities can be a treasure trove of resources—recipes that fit within various fasting windows, strategies for managing social engagements and hunger pangs, and insights into the latest research on fasting and health.

By weaving the thread of community support into the fabric of your fasting journey, you enrich your experience and contribute to a larger tapestry of collective empowerment and wellness. This shared journey, illuminated by the stories and support of others, underscores the profound impact of connection on the road to health and vitality.

Listening to Your Body: Recognizing Hunger vs. Habits

Distinguishing hunger signals

Embarking on the fasting journey invites a deeper communion with your body. This dialogue unfolds in the silence of abstention. Central to this conversation is distinguishing between true hunger and the habitual cues that often masquerade as hunger—those prompted by boredom, stress, or emotion. For women, mastering this distinction is not just about enhancing the effectiveness of fasting; it's about cultivating a profound understanding and respect for the body's authentic needs.

True hunger communicates the body's genuine need for nourishment, a physical sensation that grows gradually and can be satisfied with various foods. It's an invitation from the body to replenish and nourish, distinct from the immediate, often specific cravings triggered by habits or emotions. Recognizing this difference requires mindfulness and a willingness to pause, to inquire within, before automatically reaching for food.

Listening to your body during your fasting journey teaches you to respond to its signals with intention rather than impulse. It's a practice of tuning into the subtle cues, distinguishing between the emptiness that signals true hunger and the emotional or habitual desires for food. This awareness transforms eating from a habitual response to a conscious choice, deepening the fasting experience into a journey of self-discovery and alignment with your body's natural rhythms.

Embracing this level of attunement empowers women to navigate their fasting journey with grace, understanding that every hunger cue is not a call to eat but an opportunity to connect more deeply with themselves and their needs. This journey of differentiation between hunger and habits paves the way for a healthier, more mindful relationship with food and self.

Mindful eating practices

In the harmonious dance of fasting and nourishment, mindful eating practices emerge as a melody that enriches the fasting journey, elevating the experience from mere abstention to a profound celebration of presence and awareness. For women, incorporating mindfulness into eating practices during their windows of nourishment transforms meals into moments of deep connection with their body's signals of hunger and fullness, fostering a relationship with food rooted in intention and gratitude.

Mindful eating encourages a gentle pause, a space to breathe and truly engage with eating—savoring each bite, noticing textures, flavors, and aromas, and, most importantly, tuning into the body's cues of satisfaction and satiety. It's about eating slowly, without the distraction of screens or stress, allowing for a dialogue between body and mind that honors hunger and recognizes fullness.

This practice enhances the physical benefits of fasting by preventing overeating during feeding windows and cultivates a sense of mindfulness that spills over into other areas of life. Women learn to approach their meals—and their fasting periods—with a sense of reverence and self-care, acknowledging that each bite is an opportunity to nourish the body and the soul.

By weaving mindful eating practices into the fabric of the fasting journey, women create a tapestry of wellness rich with awareness, self-compassion, and a deepened connection to the intuitive wisdom of their bodies. This mindful approach to eating, embraced within the sacred pause of fasting, becomes a pathway to holistic health, where nourishment is received with gratitude, and every meal becomes an act of self-love.

Adapting Fasting Based on Feedback

As you journey through the landscapes of fasting, your body serves as a compass, offering feedback and signals that guide your path. This dialogue between body and practice is foundational, especially for women, as it honors the fluidity of their physiological needs across different life stages and daily rhythms. Adapting fasting lengths and eating windows in response to your body's cues is not merely a strategy; it's an act of deep listening and respect for the body's innate wisdom.

When you notice sustained energy, improved focus, or a sense of well-being signals, you affirm that your fasting regimen aligns with your body's needs. Conversely, feelings of lethargy, irritability, or overwhelming hunger are cues to reevaluate and adjust your fasting approach. Shortening the fasting window or shifting the eating period to a different time of day can restore balance and harmony.

This adaptive approach encourages a personalized fasting journey responsive to your body's needs. It empowers women to become attuned to their physiological feedback, using it as a guide to refine their fasting practices. By adjusting lengths and windows based on this feedback, fasting becomes a flexible health and vitality tool tailored to support your body's changing needs over time.

Embracing this responsive way of fasting fosters a nurturing relationship with your body, where adjustments are made with compassion and mindfulness. This approach ensures that fasting remains a supportive, enriching practice that enhances your well-being at every stage of your journey.

Navigating challenges

Navigating the challenges of hunger pangs, cravings, and social eating situations with grace and strategy is a pivotal aspect of the fasting journey for women. These moments test resilience but can become opportunities for empowerment and growth when approached with intention and understanding. The key lies in cultivating strategies that honor your fasting commitment while nurturing your well-being.

Managing Hunger Pangs and Cravings:

- **Stay Hydrated**: Often, the body can confuse signals of thirst with hunger. Drinking water, herbal teas, or a warm broth can soothe hunger without breaking your fast.
- **Mindful Breathing**: A brief mindful breathing exercise can help manage cravings by shifting focus and reducing stress, often triggering emotional eating.

Navigating Social Eating:

- **Plan Ahead**: If possible, schedule social gatherings around your eating windows or choose venues that offer flexibility in meal timing.
- **Communicate**: Sharing your fasting journey with friends and family can garner support and understanding, making it easier to navigate social situations without pressure to eat.
- **Find Alternatives**: In social settings, focusing on non-food aspects of the gathering, like engaging in conversations or enjoying the ambiance, can help divert attention from eating.

Adopting these strategies requires a blend of self-compassion and determination, recognizing that each challenge on the fasting path is a step towards deeper self-awareness and mastery. By facing these moments with preparedness and grace, women can confidently navigate the complexities of fasting, ensuring their journey is fulfilling and aligned with their wellness goals.

Hydration and Nutrient Focus During Fasting Windows

The Importance of Hydration

Hydration transcends its usual importance in fasting, becoming an essential strategy for sustaining health and enhancing the fasting experience. For women especially, understanding and prioritizing hydration is pivotal. It ensures the body remains resilient and vibrant, capable of harnessing the full benefits of fasting.

Water, the quintessence of life, should be your constant companion through-out fasting periods. It plays a critical role in metabolic functions, helps eliminate toxins, and can significantly alleviate the sensation of hunger that often accompanies fasting. Herbal teas offer a soothing alternative with diverse flavors and health benefits. They can calm the mind, aid digestion, and support overall well-being without disrupting the fast. These teas and minimal black coffee, which provide a modest caffeine boost and antioxidants, offer ways to diversify your fluid intake while maintaining the fast's integrity.

The inclusion of electrolytes is equally crucial. They are the unsung heroes that support cellular function, energy production, and the balance of fluids in your body. During longer fasting windows, when you might be more susceptible to imbalances, electrolytes can be a lifeline, helping to prevent dehydration and ensure your body's systems operate smoothly.

Incorporating a mindful approach to hydration — through water, herbal teas, minimal black coffee, and a careful balance of electrolytes — is not just about quenching thirst; it's about nurturing your body's needs, enhancing your fasting journey and embracing a holistic approach to health. This atten-tion to hydration signifies a commitment to caring for oneself, supporting the body's natural processes, and optimizing the fasting experience for longevity and vitality.

Nutrient-Dense Foods

Navigating the fasting journey with grace and wisdom involves the timing of meals and their composition. For women, choosing nutrient-dense foods during eating windows becomes a cornerstone of success, ensuring that every bite contributes to a tapestry of well-being, vitality, and longevity. This approach champions foods that are not merely calories but vessels of nourishment, packed with vitamins, minerals, antioxidants, and fiber, which collectively support the body's myriad functions, from cellular repair to immune strength.

The emphasis on whole foods — vibrant fruits, verdant vegetables, lean proteins, wholesome grains, and healthy fats — is more than a dietary choice; it affirms life's vitality. These foods work in harmony with the body's natural rhythms, enhancing the benefits of fasting by replenishing essential nutrients and optimizing bodily functions. For women, this mindful selection aids in balancing hormones, supporting reproductive health, and maintaining bone density while also offering the energy needed to thrive in daily activities.

Incorporating nutrient-rich foods into meals transforms the eating window from a mere break in the fast into a celebration of nourishment. It's an opportunity to fuel the body thoughtfully and lovingly with foods that resonate with its intrinsic needs, elevating the fasting experience from a routine to a ritual of self-care and respect. This deliberate choice to nourish deeply supports the physical body and cultivates a mindset of abundance and gratitude, essential ingredients for a fulfilling fasting journey and a vibrant, healthful life.

Supplementation Considerations

Embarking on fasting, especially during extended periods, invites exploration into the world of supplementation, a journey that complements the fasting experience with a tapestry of nutritional support. This becomes particularly poignant for women as their bodies navigate the ebb and flow of nutritional needs against the backdrop of fasting. Thoughtful supplementation can gracefully fill the dietary gaps, ensuring the body remains a wellspring of vitality and resilience.

When to Consider Supplementation:

- Amid longer fasts, when daily intake of essential nutrients might not meet the body's requirements.
- To address specific dietary limitations or preferences that might result in gaps, such as plant-based diets lacking B12, iron, and particular omega-3s.
- To support particular health considerations unique to women, including bone density through calcium and vitamin D, and hormonal health with targeted support like magnesium and vitamin B6.

Guidance on Supplement Usage:

- Engage with a healthcare professional to tailor your supplement strategy to your individual health needs and fasting practices, ensuring a harmonious integration with your lifestyle and wellness objectives.
- Prioritize high-quality supplements, favoring those derived from whole-food sources for better absorption and efficacy.
- Consider the timing of supplementation, aligning intake with eating windows when possible to optimize nutrient absorption and benefit.

By weaving supplements into the fabric of your fasting regimen with intention and care, you provide your body with a robust foundation of support. This strategic approach ensures that each step on your fasting journey is taken with strength, nourished by a spectrum of essential nutrients that fortify your path toward health and vitality.

Medication consideration

Navigating the terrain of medication intake during fasting periods requires a delicate balance, particularly for women, who may encounter unique challenges and considerations in synchronizing their medication regimen with fasting schedules. This interplay between fasting and medication is not just about timing; it's about understanding the body's nuanced responses and ensuring health and safety remain at the forefront of your fasting journey.

Critical Considerations for Medication During Fasting:

- **Absorption and Efficacy**: Some medications require food to be adequately absorbed or to mitigate potential side effects, such as gastrointestinal discomfort. The absence of food during fasting windows can alter the medication's effectiveness and the body's response to it.
- **Blood Sugar Levels**: For women managing diabetes or blood sugar concerns, fasting can significantly impact glucose levels, necessitating a careful approach to medication timing and monitoring to prevent hypoglycemia.
- **Hormonal Medications**: Women on hormonal treatments, including contraceptives or hormone replacement therapy, should consult healthcare providers to understand how fasting might affect hormonal balance and medication effectiveness.

Navigating Medication Intake:

- Engage in open dialogue with a healthcare provider, discussing your fasting intentions and seeking advice on adjusting medication schedules or dosages as needed.
- Monitor your body's response closely. Fasting introduces changes to your body's rhythm, which could necessitate adjustments to medication timing to align with eating windows or to ensure optimal efficacy and safety.
- Consider the type of fasting regimen you're following. Shorter intermittent fasting windows offer more flexibility for medication intake than extended fasts.

Embarking on a fasting journey as a woman, especially when medication is part of your daily regimen, underscores the importance of personalized care and informed decision-making. Through careful planning and professional guidance, you can navigate these waters safely, ensuring that your fasting experience supports your health goals and medical needs.

Balancing Macronutrients

In pursuing a fulfilling fasting experience, understanding the art of macronutrient balance becomes a cornerstone of success, especially for women who seek to sustain their energy levels and promote a sense of fullness throughout their fasting and eating windows. The symphony of proteins, fats, and carbohydrates is pivotal in nourishing the body, supporting metabolic health, and ensuring every meal is a step toward wellness.

Harmonizing Macronutrients:

- **Proteins**: The building blocks of life, proteins are crucial for muscle repair, hormonal health, and satiety. Including various protein sources, such as lean meats, fish, legumes, and dairy, supports physical strength and helps manage hunger pangs during fasting periods.
- **Fats**: Healthy fats, found in avocados, nuts, seeds, and olive oil, provide sustained energy and are essential for absorbing fat-soluble vitamins. Incorporating these into your diet enhances meal satisfaction and supports cognitive function.
- **Carbohydrates**: Choosing complex carbohydrates like whole grains, vegetables, and fruits ensures a steady release of energy, fiber for digestive health, and vital nutrients. This mindful selection aids in maintaining blood sugar levels and provides the necessary fuel for your body's daily functions.

For women embarking on a fasting journey, balancing these macronutrients is not just about dietary compliance; it's about creating nourishing and satisfying meals, ensuring that your body is well-equipped to thrive during fasting and beyond. This holistic approach to macronutrient balance fosters a sustainable, health-promoting fasting experience, allowing you to embrace the benefits of fasting with vigor and vitality.

Chapter 3: Fasting and the Menstrual Cycle

Syncing Your Fast with Your Cycle

Understanding your cycle
Navigating the ebb and flow of menstrual cycles is an essential aspect of fasting for women, offering profound insights into the body's hormonal landscape. Understanding the nuances of each phase—follicular, ovulatory, luteal, and menstrual—unveils opportunities to align fasting practices with the body's intrinsic rhythms, enhancing well-being and optimizing results.

Harmonizing Fasting with Hormonal Cycles:

- **Follicular Phase**: Post-menstruation, when energy levels rise and estrogen begins to surge, might be an opportune time to engage in more rigorous fasting or intense physical activity, leveraging the body's natural inclinations for growth and renewal.
- **Ovulatory Phase**: Marked by a peak in fertility and a further increase in estrogen, this phase can bring about heightened energy and mood. Fasting during this time may feel more manageable, and the body's metabolic responses are primed for optimal performance.
- **Luteal Phase**: As the body prepares for the possibility of pregnancy, energy expenditure increases, and cravings may arise. Gentle fasting

approaches or shorter fasting windows can accommodate the body's increased nutritional needs and energy demands.

· **Menstrual Phase**: During menstruation, when energy may wane, and the body seeks restoration, listening closely to its cues is beneficial. Adjusting fasting intensity and focusing on nourishment and hydration can support the body's healing processes.

For women, intertwining the knowledge of menstrual cycles with fasting fosters a deeper connection with their bodies and empowers them to tailor fasting practices to their unique hormonal landscapes. This mindful approach ensures that fasting supports holistic health, honoring the body's rhythms and needs throughout the cycle.

Fasting Phases Alignment

Aligning fasting methods with the follicular and luteal phases of the menstrual cycle can significantly enhance women's hormonal balance, overall health, and well-being. This tailored approach respects the body's natural rhythms, leveraging the unique hormonal fluctuations during these phases to optimize fasting benefits.

Follicular Phase Alignment:

The follicular phase, beginning after menstruation and lasting until ovu-lation, is characterized by rising estrogen levels. This phase allows women to engage in more aggressive or extended fasting strategies. The increase in estrogen promotes energy utilization and mood elevation, making it an ideal time to capitalize on more stringent fasting methods like the 16/8 method or even occasional 24-hour fasts. This synchronization can improve metabolic flexibility, increase fat loss, and enhance cognitive function.

Luteal Phase Considerations:

The luteal phase follows ovulation and is marked by increased progesterone, preparing the body for potential pregnancy. This phase often involves heightened emotional sensitivities, cravings, and a higher basal metabolic rate. During this period, shorter fasting windows or more nourishing, less restrictive fasting approaches, such as the 12/12 method, can support the body's increased energy and nutritional needs. Adapting fasting practices to accommodate these changes helps manage cravings, maintain energy levels, and support emotional well-being.

Aligning fasting with the menstrual cycle's phases allows for a harmonious balance between fasting benefits and hormonal health. It acknowledges the body's changing needs throughout the cycle, enhancing the efficacy of fasting without compromising nutritional support. This personalized approach minimizes potential stressors on the hormonal system, ensuring that fasting supports rather than disrupts menstrual regularity and hormonal balance. Furthermore, it empowers women to feel more in tune with their bodies, fostering a positive and nurturing fasting experience that aligns with their physiological and emotional states throughout the month.

Adaptive Fasting Techniques

Adaptive fasting techniques present a nuanced approach that allows women to adjust the intensity and duration of their fasting periods to align with the various stages of their menstrual cycle, thereby supporting overall well-being. This method acknowledges the body's fluctuating hormonal needs and adapts fasting practices accordingly, ensuring that women can harness the benefits of fasting without compromising their health.

During the follicular phase, which spans from the end of menstruation to ovulation, women may have higher energy levels and increased metabolic flexibility due to rising estrogen levels. This is an opportune time to engage in more rigorous fasting methods, such as longer fasts or strict time-restricted eating windows, which can enhance fat loss, improve mental clarity, and boost energy.

As the cycle progresses into the luteal phase, characterized by higher progesterone levels and premenstrual symptoms, the body's energy and nutritional needs increase. Reducing fasting intensity is advisable if changes are needed by shortening fasting periods or adopting more lenient fasting windows. This adjustment helps manage cravings, supports emotional well-being, and sustains energy levels, acknowledging the body's need for increased nutritional support during this phase.

Adaptive fasting techniques thus encourage a flexible, cyclic approach to fasting that respects the body's natural rhythms. By tuning into and honoring these physiological cues, women can create a fasting schedule that supports hormonal balance, optimizes health outcomes, and enhances their overall fasting experience. This approach promotes physical well-being and fosters a deeper connection with one's body, empowering women to make informed, supportive choices throughout their menstrual cycle.

Cycle tracking tools

Incorporating cycle-tracking tools into your wellness routine offers a personalized approach to understanding and aligning with your body's unique rhythms, especially when integrating fasting into your lifestyle. Leveraging technology through apps or maintaining a traditional journal can significantly enhance your ability to plan and adjust your fasting schedule in harmony with the phases of your menstrual cycle, ultimately optimizing your health and fasting outcomes.

Cycle tracking apps provide a convenient and precise way to monitor your menstrual cycle, predicting ovulation and menstruation phases with remarkable accuracy. By inputting daily symptoms, energy levels, and other relevant health markers, these apps can offer insights into your hormonal fluctuations and how they might impact your fasting experience. This data becomes invaluable when planning your fasting intensity and duration, allowing for adjustments that respect your body's changing needs throughout the month.

Similarly, keeping a journal dedicated to tracking your menstrual cycle alongside your fasting schedules and experiences offers a more personalized touch. It lets you note patterns over time, such as how your hunger levels, energy, and mood correlate with different cycle phases. This reflective practice not only aids in tailoring your fasting approach but also deepens your connection with your body, fostering a holistic understanding of how fasting affects your physical and emotional well-being across your menstrual cycle.

These cycle-tracking tools empower you with knowledge, enabling a more nuanced and effective fasting plan that aligns with your body's natural rhythms. This personalized planning approach supports hormonal balance, enhances the benefits of fasting, and contributes to a more fulfilling and sustainable fasting journey.

Managing Energy Levels and Cravings

Energy Fluctuations

Understanding and managing energy levels and cravings are crucial for women who integrate fasting into their lifestyle, especially concerning the menstrual cycle's ebb and flow. Recognizing the natural fluctuations in energy and appetite throughout the cycle can significantly inform how one might adjust fasting schedules for optimal well-being and effectiveness.

During the menstrual cycle, hormonal shifts can significantly impact energy levels and cravings. For instance, the follicular phase, particularly right after menstruation, often increases energy and mood, making it more suitable for extended or intense fasting periods. Conversely, the luteal phase, which precedes menstruation, might see a dip in energy and increased cravings. This suggests that shorter fasting windows or more lenient fasting methods may be more appropriate to accommodate the body's heightened nutritional and emotional needs.

By identifying these patterns, women can tailor their fasting schedules to align with their body's signals, optimizing energy levels and managing cravings more effectively. This approach enhances the fasting experience and supports overall health and hormonal balance. It acknowledges the body's innate wisdom and adapts to its changing needs, ensuring that fasting remains a supportive and sustainable practice throughout the different phases of the menstrual cycle.

Incorporating mindful eating practices during eating windows, focusing on nutrient-dense foods that satisfy and nourish, can further support energy levels and help manage cravings. By listening to their bodies and adjusting fasting and eating practices accordingly, women can navigate the challenges of fluctuating energy and cravings gracefully and easily, making fasting a more enjoyable and beneficial part of their health regimen.

Craving Control

Managing cravings is a pivotal aspect of a successful fasting journey, especially for women navigating the intricate balance of their hormonal landscape. By implementing strategic approaches during eating windows and adopting mindful eating practices, women can significantly enhance their ability to control cravings and maintain their fasting regimen without feeling deprived or overwhelmed.

Focusing on nutrient-dense food choices during eating periods is fundamental. A diet rich in whole foods such as vegetables, fruits, lean proteins, healthy fats, and whole grains can provide the body with essential vitamins, minerals, and fiber. These nutrients support overall health and well-being and play a crucial role in stabilizing blood sugar levels and satiety, which can reduce cravings. For instance, foods high in protein and fiber are particularly effective at promoting feelings of fullness for more extended periods, helping curb the desire to snack unnecessarily.

Mindful eating practices further empower women to manage cravings by fostering a deeper connection with their hunger and fullness cues. By eating slowly and without distraction, women can better recognize when they are hungry versus when they might reach for food due to boredom, stress, or emotional reasons. This awareness can lead to more intentional food choices during eating windows and reduce impulsive eating behaviors.

Staying hydrated by drinking water and herbal teas and incorporating minimal black coffee can also help manage hunger and cravings. Sometimes, the body may signal hunger when it is dehydrated. Women can better differentiate between true hunger and thirst by ensuring adequate hydration, further aiding in craving control.

Incorporating these strategies—focusing on nutrient-dense foods, practicing mindful eating, and staying hydrated—allows women to navigate their fasting journey more efficiently and successfully. By being conscious of their body's needs and responding appropriately, women can effectively manage cravings, making fasting a more enjoyable and sustainable lifestyle.

Supplementation Guidance

Within the nuanced tapestry of fasting, especially for women attuned to the rhythms of their menstrual cycle, supplementation can play a supportive role, enhancing energy levels and mitigating cravings during specific cycle phases. Thoughtful supplementation, aligned with the body's changing needs, offers a foundation of support, ensuring that fasting becomes a journey of empowerment and well-being.

During the follicular phase, when energy begins to ascend, supplements like B vitamins can bolster vitality, supporting the body's natural energy production processes. Magnesium, too, plays a dual role: it can enhance sleep quality, thereby indirectly boosting energy levels and alleviating cravings, particularly those for sweets, by regulating blood sugar levels and supporting insulin sensitivity.

As the cycle progresses into the luteal phase, where cravings and energy fluctuations become more pronounced, omega-3 fatty acids emerge as valuable allies. These supplements support mood and cognitive function and help manage cravings by promoting a sense of satiety and well-being. Additionally, incorporating vitamin D and calcium during this phase can keep hormonal balance and overall mood, further aiding craving control and energy maintenance.

By integrating these supplements into their fasting regimen, women can navigate the ebbs and flows of their menstrual cycle with greater ease and resilience. It's essential, however, to consult with a healthcare provider before beginning any supplementation, ensuring that it complements your fasting practice and health goals. Tailoring supplement choices to the body's cyclical needs enhances the fasting experience and supports a holistic approach to health and vitality, empowering women to thrive throughout their fasting journey.

Stress Management

In fasting, particularly for women, the interplay between stress management and regulating energy and cravings is pivotal. Acknowledging and addressing stress is not just about enhancing mental well-being; it's about creating a conducive environment for fasting that supports the body's physiological needs and goals.

Stress, often a silent saboteur, can significantly impact energy levels and elicit cravings, making fasting more challenging. Cortisol, the stress hormone, not only influences appetite but can also prompt the body to store fat, especially around the midsection. Thus, incorporating stress reduction techniques becomes essential in fasting to maintain energy, manage cravings, and support overall health.

Mindfulness practices, including meditation and deep-breathing exercises, emerge as powerful fasting tools. By fostering a sense of calm and presence, these practices can help mitigate the body's stress response, thereby reducing cortisol levels. This stress reduction can directly influence cravings, making them more manageable and lessening the likelihood of fasting disruptions.

Moreover, adapting fasting schedules to stress levels can be incredibly beneficial. Shortening fasting windows or opting for gentler fasting methods can help the body better manage energy requirements and cravings during high stress. This adaptive approach not only honors the body's current state but also supports long-term sustainability and success in fasting.

Integrating stress management techniques and making appropriate fasting adjustments in response to stress levels are crucial strategies. They enhance the fasting experience and empower women to navigate their fasting journey with grace, resilience, and a deeper connection to their body's needs.

Fasting Strategies for Menstrual Health

Symptom Mitigation

In the tapestry of women's health, fasting emerges as a tool for weight management or metabolic enhancement and a potential ally in alleviating common menstrual symptoms. Bloating, fatigue, and mood swings, often unwelcome yet frequent visitors during the menstrual cycle, can significantly impact daily life and overall well-being. Fasting, with its myriad benefits, offers a promising avenue for symptom mitigation, presenting a holistic approach to managing these menstrual challenges.

By regulating blood sugar levels and improving hormonal balance, fasting can play a pivotal role in reducing bloating, a common complaint among many women premenstrually. This reduction in bloating is a matter of physical comfort and contributes to a sense of lightness and well-being. Furthermore, fasting can enhance energy levels by improving insulin sensitivity and facilitating a more efficient fuel utilization process. This shift in energy metabolism may help counteract the fatigue that often accompanies the menstrual cycle.

Mood swings, another prevalent symptom, may also see improvement through fasting. The practice can aid in stabilizing mood by influencing neurotransmitter function and promoting a balanced hormonal landscape. The psychological benefits of fasting, including increased mental clarity and a sense of achievement, can further bolster emotional well-being during this time.

Thus, when approached thoughtfully and tailored to individual needs, fasting can offer women a powerful strategy for mitigating the physical and emotional symptoms associated with their menstrual cycle, enhancing their quality of life, and empowering them in their health journeys.

Inflammatory Response

Fasting harbors the potential to be a transformative ally in menstrual health, particularly its impact on inflammation, a critical factor that can exacerbate menstrual symptoms and discomfort. Fasting initiates a cascade of cellular and molecular events that can significantly reduce inflammation, offering a beacon of relief for many women.

The mechanism behind fasting's anti-inflammatory effects is multifaceted, involving reducing pro-inflammatory cytokines and enhancing cellular autophagy. This process, where cells cleanse themselves of damaged components, can reduce systemic inflammation. For women, this reduction in inflammation can translate into less severe menstrual symptoms, as inflammation is a known contributor to cramps, bloating, and general discomfort.

Moreover, fasting's role in regulating hormone levels further complements its anti-inflammatory benefits. By improving insulin sensitivity and reducing insulin-like growth factor 1 (IGF-1) levels, fasting can help balance other hormones, including estrogen and progesterone, which play pivotal roles in menstrual health. This hormonal balance reduces menstrual discomfort and improves overall reproductive health.

The benefits of incorporating fasting into a woman's health regimen extend beyond weight loss or metabolic health; they reach into the essence of menstrual well-being. By mitigating inflammation, fasting offers a pathway to alleviate common menstrual symptoms. It paves the way for a more balanced, vibrant health, empowering women to navigate their menstrual cycles more efficiently and comfortably.

Hormonal Regulation

Fasting emerges as a compelling approach to fostering hormonal harmony, offering a natural avenue for women to mitigate the symptoms of hormonal imbalances. This practice, steeped in ancient traditions and validated by modern science, taps into the body's intrinsic mechanisms for self-regulation and healing, providing a foundation for enhanced well-being and hormonal equilibrium.

At the heart of fasting's appeal is its capacity to modulate insulin levels, a pivotal hormone that influences various bodily functions, including other hormone productions. By improving insulin sensitivity, fasting can indirectly support the balance of sex hormones such as estrogen and progesterone, critical to menstrual health, fertility, and mood regulation. This balance is essential for minimizing symptoms associated with hormonal imbalances, such as irregular periods, mood swings, and acne.

Furthermore, fasting can elevate human growth hormone (HGH) levels, vital to health and longevity. Increased HGH levels contribute to improved metabolism, muscle strength, and fat loss, further supporting hormonal balance by reducing the risk of conditions like PCOS, often linked to insulin resistance.

By initiating these physiological changes, fasting not only aids in directly managing hormonal imbalances but also enhances overall health, providing a holistic approach to well-being. For women navigating the challenges of hormonal fluctuations, fasting offers a promising strategy to regain balance, reduce symptoms, and embrace a more harmonious state of health.

Personalized Fasting Plans

Crafting a personalized fasting plan is paramount for women who seek to address their unique menstrual health concerns and achieve specific wellness goals. This bespoke approach acknowledges the intricate dance of hormones that governs a woman's cycle, offering a tailored strategy to harness the benefits of fasting in alignment with her body's rhythms and needs.

The cornerstone of a personalized fasting plan lies in its adaptability, allowing for adjustments based on menstrual cycle phases, symptoms, and lifestyle demands. For instance, a woman may find a gentler, shorter fasting regimen supportive during the luteal phase when energy levels and cravings might fluctuate, transitioning to more extended fasting periods in the follicular phase when energy is abundant and hormonal balance is more stable.

Incorporating personal health goals into the fasting plan is equally vital. Whether aiming for weight management, improved energy, or reduced menstrual symptoms, the fasting regimen can be fine-tuned to optimize results. This might mean varying fasting durations, experimenting with different fasting windows, or integrating specific dietary focuses during eating periods to support hormonal health, such as increased phytoestrogens or anti-inflammatory foods.

Ultimately, a personalized fasting plan empowers women to take an active role in their health, providing a framework that respects and responds to their body's signals. Through careful planning and ongoing adjustment, women can discover the fasting approach that resonates with their body's needs, unlocking the potential for enhanced menstrual health and overall well-being.

The Impact of Fasting on Fertility and PCOS

Fertility Considerations

Embarking on a fasting journey entails mindful consideration of its impact on fertility, making it essential for women contemplating conception to understand how fasting practices might influence their reproductive health. Fasting, with its myriad health benefits, can also affect hormonal balance and menstrual cycles, factors integral to fertility.

For women aiming to conceive, the timing and intensity of fasting require careful calibration. During pre-conception, moderate fasting enhances fertility by improving overall health, reducing inflammation, and balancing hormones. However, overly restrictive fasting or fasting for extended periods could disrupt menstrual regularity and ovulation, crucial elements for conception.

Women should adopt a more lenient fasting regimen in the months leading up to conception attempts, focusing on nourishing the body and maintaining a stable hormonal environment conducive to fertility. This might include shorter fasting windows and ensuring that eating periods are rich in fertility-supporting nutrients.

Moreover, once the journey towards conception begins, pausing or significantly adjusting fasting practices can provide the body with the consistent energy and nutritional support needed for ovulation and early pregnancy stages.

In summary, while fasting can be a powerful tool for health enhancement, women considering fertility must navigate their fasting practices with an attuned awareness of their body's cues and modify their approach to support the best possible foundation for conception.

PCOS Management

Polycystic Ovary Syndrome (PCOS) presents a complex challenge for many women, characterized by irregular menstrual cycles, ovulation issues, and insulin resistance, among other symptoms. Fasting emerges as a promising strategy to manage PCOS, offering a pathway to mitigate symptoms and enhance ovulatory function through its impact on hormonal balance and metabolic health.

Intermittent fasting can improve insulin sensitivity, a crucial factor for women with PCOS. By extending the periods without food intake, fasting encourages the body to utilize glucose more efficiently, potentially reducing insulin levels and alleviating one of the core disturbances of PCOS. This improved insulin sensitivity can lead to more regular menstrual cycles and improved ovulation, critical outcomes for women facing fertility challenges linked to PCOS.

Moreover, fasting can aid in weight management, a common concern for those with PCOS. Excess weight often exacerbates PCOS symptoms, and the weight loss associated with consistent fasting practices can lead to a reduction in symptoms, including improved hormonal profiles and an increased likelihood of ovulation.

However, women with PCOS must approach fasting with caution and under medical guidance. Tailoring the fasting regimen to individual health status, lifestyle, and nutritional needs ensures that fasting acts as a beneficial tool rather than a stressor, promoting overall well-being and reproductive health.

Insulin Sensitivity Improvement

Fasting holds transformative potential for women, particularly in improving insulin sensitivity, a cornerstone in managing conditions like Polycystic Ovary Syndrome (PCOS) and enhancing fertility. Insulin sensitivity refers to the body's ability to use insulin to lower blood sugar levels efficiently, a process often impaired in PCOS. This impairment can lead to elevated insulin and blood sugar levels, contributing to a range of symptoms, including weight gain, irregular menstrual cycles, and fertility issues.

By adopting intermittent fasting, women can significantly impact their insulin sensitivity. During fasting, the body switches from glucose to fat as its primary energy source, requiring less insulin. This reduction in the demand for insulin over time can help restore the body's natural insulin sensitivity. For women with PCOS, this improvement can mean not only a reduction in PCOS symptoms but also enhanced chances of conception due to more regular ovulation and balanced hormone levels.

Moreover, fasting-induced weight loss further enhances insulin sensitivity. Excess body fat around the abdomen is linked to increased insulin resistance. By facilitating weight management, fasting contributes to a more favorable hormonal environment for ovulation and fertility.

It's essential, however, for women to approach fasting with awareness and adapt it to their unique health profiles. Consulting with healthcare professionals ensures that fasting is integrated into their lifestyle to support their health and fertility goals without compromising nutritional balance.

Fasting and Reproductive Health Research

In women's health, the intersection of fasting and reproductive health garners increasing scientific attention. Emerging research offers intriguing insights into how fasting may influence fertility and the management of Poly-cystic Ovary Syndrome (PCOS), a common condition affecting reproductive health.

Studies suggest that fasting, particularly intermittent fasting, can positively impact hormonal balance, which is crucial for reproductive health. For women with PCOS, characterized by insulin resistance and hormonal imbalances, fasting can be particularly beneficial. The practice has been shown to improve insulin sensitivity, reduce insulin levels, and aid in weight loss—all factors that can help regulate menstrual cycles and improve ovulatory function. These changes are vital for enhancing fertility in women with PCOS, who often struggle with irregular ovulation.

Furthermore, research indicates fasting can positively affect hormones such as leptin and adiponectin, which are involved in hunger and fat storage regulation. Adjustments in these hormones can lead to better metabolic health and potentially improve fertility outcomes.

However, the scientific community also emphasizes the need for personalized fasting approaches, especially regarding reproductive health. While the data is promising, individual differences mean that fasting's effectiveness can vary. Ongoing studies explore these dynamics, underscoring the importance of consulting healthcare providers to tailor fasting practices to one's health profile and fertility goals. This evolving research landscape encourages a cautious yet hopeful perspective on fasting as a tool for enhancing reproductive health and managing PCOS.

Chapter 4: Fasting Through Menopause

Understanding Menopause and Metabolic Health

Menopause Overview
Menopause marks a significant phase in a woman's life, characterized by the cessation of menstrual cycles and the end of reproductive capability. This transition typically occurs between 45 and 55 but can vary widely among individuals. Menopause is not an overnight event but a gradual process that unfolds through several stages, beginning with perimenopause, transitioning into menopause, and culminating in postmenopause.

Perimenopause is the precursor to menopause, during which a woman's body starts to make less estrogen. This stage can last for several years, during which women might experience irregular menstrual cycles, hot flashes, sleep disturbances, and mood swings. Menopause is confirmed when a woman has not had a menstrual cycle for 12 consecutive months. Following this, she enters postmenopause, which lasts for the rest of her life.

These stages bring about significant metabolic changes, primarily due to the decline in estrogen levels. Reduced estrogen can affect body composition, leading to increased abdominal fat and a higher risk for cardiovascular diseases and osteoporosis. The metabolic slowdown associated with aging also means energy needs decrease, making weight management more challenging.

Understanding these changes is crucial for managing health during and after the transition. By recognizing the signs and stages of menopause, women can better prepare for the metabolic shifts accompanying this natural phase of life, adopting lifestyle and dietary practices supporting overall well-being during these transformative years.

Fasting's Role in Metabolic Adaptation

During the menopausal transition, women face various metabolic challenges, including changes in body composition, slowed metabolism, and increased risk for chronic conditions like type 2 diabetes and cardiovascular disease. Fasting is a powerful tool to support metabolic health during this period, offering a pathway to adapt and respond positively to these changes.

Fasting can enhance metabolic flexibility—the body's ability to switch between burning glucose and fat for energy—thereby improving insulin sensitivity and aiding in weight management. This adaptability is particularly beneficial as estrogen levels decline and insulin resistance becomes more common. By incorporating fasting into their lifestyle, women can help offset the metabolic slowdown experienced during menopause, facilitating weight control and reducing the risk of metabolic syndrome.

Moreover, fasting promotes autophagy, the body's mechanism for cleaning out damaged cells and regenerating new ones, which can decline with age. This process is vital for maintaining healthy cellular function and can improve overall health and longevity.

By strategically utilizing fasting during the menopausal transition, women can support their body's natural adaptation processes, helping to maintain metabolic health, enhance energy levels, and protect against age-related diseases.

Hormonal fluctuations

Menopause signifies a pivotal time in a woman's life, characterized by significant hormonal fluctuations, particularly in estrogen and progesterone levels. These changes can lead to a host of symptoms, including hot flashes, night sweats, mood swings, and weight gain. Fasting offers a promising avenue for managing these hormonal imbalances, potentially easing menopause-related discomfort.

Fasting can influence hormonal activity by enhancing insulin sensitivity and lowering insulin levels, which, in turn, may help in balancing other hormones affected by insulin regulation, such as estrogen and progesterone. Moreover, fasting promotes the release of human growth hormone (HGH), which plays a role in maintaining muscle mass and metabolic rate. Both are crucial during the menopausal transition when muscle mass decreases, and the metabolic rate slows down.

By incorporating fasting strategies, women can potentially mitigate some of the metabolic and hormonal challenges associated with menopause. It can lead to a more balanced hormonal environment, alleviating some common symptoms and contributing to well-being during this transformative phase of life. However, women need to approach fasting with mindfulness and possibly under the guidance of a healthcare professional to ensure it aligns with their health status and goals.

Longevity and Quality of Life

The golden years post-menopause offer a unique opportunity for women to focus on longevity and quality of life. Fasting is a powerful tool in this pursuit, potentially extending lifespan and enhancing life's quality by promoting health and vitality. Studies suggest that fasting can stimulate autophagy, the body's way of cleaning out damaged cells, to regenerate newer, healthier ones. This process is crucial for aging gracefully, as it can help delay the onset of age-related diseases and conditions.

Moreover, fasting has been linked to improved brain health, including enhanced cognitive function and a reduced risk of neurodegenerative diseases. For women navigating the post-menopausal phase, this is particularly compelling, offering a strategy to maintain mental acuity and emotional balance.

Incorporating fasting into one's lifestyle could also lead to better metabolic health, reduced inflammation, and improved cardiovascular health, all contributing to a higher quality of life. These benefits suggest that fasting is not just about adding years to life but, more importantly, adding life to years, allowing women to thrive in their later stages with vigor, clarity, and resilience.

Tailored Fasting Approaches for Menopausal Women

Identifying Suitable Fasting Methods

For menopausal women, identifying fasting methods that resonate with their unique physiological and lifestyle needs is vital to harnessing fasting's myriad benefits. This transition period demands an approach that addresses metabolic shifts and supports emotional well-being and hormonal balance.

Intermittent fasting, with its flexible nature, offers a variety of schedules that can be tailored to individual preferences and health goals. For instance, the 16/8 method, involving 16 hours of fasting followed by an 8-hour eating window, can be particularly beneficial for managing weight and improving insulin sensitivity—a common concern during menopause. This method allows for a daily rhythm that can easily be adjusted to accommodate energy levels and lifestyle demands.

The 5:2 method, where normal eating is interspersed with two days of reduced-calorie intake each week. This approach can help mitigate inflammation and support cardiovascular health without the rigidity of daily fasting.

For those seeking a gentler introduction to fasting or dealing with significant menopause-related symptoms, time-restricted eating within a 12-hour window may offer a more manageable starting point, fostering metabolic flexibility while ensuring sufficient nutrient intake.

Selecting a fasting schedule that aligns with personal health objectives and daily routines. By doing so, menopausal women can effectively utilize fasting to enhance their health, vitality, and overall quality of life during this transformative phase.

Adjusting Fasting Based on Symptoms

Navigating through menopause requires a nuanced approach to fasting sensitive to the body's changing needs and the array of symptoms that can arise. Customizing fasting plans offers a strategic way to alleviate some of the most common menopausal discomforts, such as hot flashes, sleep disturbances, and mood swings, enhancing well-being during this transition.

For instance, women experiencing severe hot flashes might find shorter fasting periods more manageable, as long periods without food can sometimes exacerbate these symptoms. Integrating a light, nutritious snack into the evening can help stabilize blood sugar levels overnight, potentially reducing night sweats and improving sleep quality.

Adjustments to the timing of the fasting window can also play a critical role in managing sleep disturbances. Finishing the last meal earlier in the evening can enhance sleep quality by allowing digestion to occur well before bedtime, thus promoting a more restful night's sleep.

Furthermore, incorporating stress-reducing practices such as gentle yoga or meditation into the fasting routine can help mitigate mood swings and improve overall emotional balance. By attentively listening to their bodies and adjusting their fasting protocols to address specific symptoms, women can navigate menopause with greater ease and comfort, making this significant life stage more manageable and less disruptive.

Integration with Lifestyle

Integrating fasting into daily life during menopause is about finding harmony between the body's evolving needs and one's lifestyle, ensuring that energy levels and social engagements are maintained without compromise. This transition period requires strategies that flexibly accommodate the fluctuating energy levels commonly experienced by menopausal women, allowing them to continue enjoying life's pleasures, including social meals and gatherings.

A key strategy is adopting a flexible fasting approach, which allows for adjustments based on daily energy needs and social calendars. On days filled with activities or events, shorter fasting windows or even intermittent fasting can ensure participation in social meals without feeling excluded or disrupting the rhythm of social interactions. This adaptability ensures that fasting enhances, rather than limits, life during menopause.

Moreover, planning fasting schedules can help manage energy levels more effectively, ensuring that the most energy-intensive tasks are aligned with eating windows when nourishment is available to fuel the body. This thoughtful synchronization between fasting, energy management, and social activities ensures that women can navigate menopause gracefully, maintaining their social bonds and vitality without letting fasting become a barrier to life's joys.

Continuous Adaptation

Continuous adaptation is the cornerstone of a successful fasting regimen during menopause, recognizing that as a woman's body navigates through this transformative phase, her fasting practices must evolve with her changing symptoms and health status. This dynamic approach ensures that fasting remains a supportive tool, enhancing well-being rather than becoming a rigid structure that disregards the body's shifting needs.

As menopausal symptoms fluctuate, from hot flashes to changes in metabolic rate, the flexibility to adjust fasting schedules, durations, and even the types of fasting becomes paramount. This might mean shortening fasting windows during periods of intense symptoms or adjusting the timing of fasts to better align with energy levels and sleep patterns.

Listening to the body's cues and being open to modifying fasting practices ensures that fasting supports hormonal balance, energy levels, and overall health. Regular check-ins with healthcare providers can also provide valuable guidance, ensuring that fasting aligns with current health needs and contributes positively to the menopausal journey. Embracing continuous adaptation in fasting practices empowers women to navigate menopause confidently, using fasting as a flexible ally in maintaining health and vitality.

Nutritional Needs During Menopause: What Changes?

Nutrient Requirements

During menopause, a woman's nutritional needs undergo significant changes, reflecting the physiological adjustments her body is experiencing. Focusing on when and what to eat during those precious eating windows becomes crucial to meet these evolving needs. As estrogen levels decline, there's an increased need for certain nutrients to support bone health, heart health, and overall well-being. Calcium, vitamin D, magnesium, and vitamin K are paramount for bone density, while omega-3 fatty acids support heart health and may help to alleviate some menopausal symptoms.

Incorporating a variety of nutrient-dense foods into eating windows becomes essential. Leafy greens, fatty fish, nuts, seeds, and whole grains can provide a rich tapestry of these vital nutrients, helping to combat the increased risk of osteoporosis and cardiovascular disease. Additionally, fiber-rich foods can aid digestion and help manage weight, a common concern during menopause due to metabolic changes.

By emphasizing the quality of food intake during eating windows, women can address the nutritional shifts of menopause, supporting their body's health and easing the transition through this natural phase of life. This strategic approach to nutrition ensures that fasting not only aids in managing weight and improving metabolic health but also fortifies the body against the specific challenges menopause presents.

Bone Health

In the journey through menopause, the significance of bone health cannot be overstated significantly, as the decline in estrogen levels increases the risk of osteoporosis. This natural phase of life requires an intensified focus on calcium and vitamin D—two pillars of bone strength. Calcium is crucial in maintaining bone density, while vitamin D enhances calcium absorption and growth. However, with fasting, ensuring adequate intake of these nutrients requires mindful planning.

For women navigating menopause, integrating calcium-rich foods like dairy products, leafy greens, and fortified foods into eating windows is vital. Similarly, sources of vitamin D, such as fatty fish, egg yolks, and sunlight exposure, are essential. Since fasting limits the time for nutrient intake, prioritizing these nutrients during eating windows becomes a strategic approach to safeguarding bone health.

Moreover, considering the body's changing ability to absorb these nutrients, supplementation may be a prudent addition to the diet, subject to a healthcare provider's guidance. This proactive focus on calcium and vitamin D intake supports bone health. It acts as a preventive measure against the increased risk of fractures, ensuring that women can approach menopause with confidence and resilience.

Heart Health

As women journey through menopause, the protective effects of estrogen wane, unveiling an increased risk of cardiovascular disease. This pivotal time underscores the importance of heart health, where fasting, paired with heart-healthy foods and practices, becomes a beacon of preventive care. Embracing a diet rich in omega-3 fatty acids, found in fish like salmon and flaxseeds, can combat inflammation and support heart health. Fruits, vegetables, whole grains, and nuts, consumed during eating windows, provide fiber, antioxidants, and healthy fats, acting as cornerstones of a heart-protective diet.

Moreover, fasting offers a unique advantage by potentially improving lipid profiles and reducing inflammation, which is closely tied to heart health. However, integrating such dietary practices must be approached with balance and mindfulness, ensuring that the body's nutritional needs are met without compromising the benefits of fasting.

Physical activity, another ally in the quest for heart health, complements fasting by enhancing cardiovascular fitness and managing weight. Together, these strategies form a holistic approach to mitigating the increased risk of heart disease during menopause, empowering women to navigate this transition with health and vitality at the forefront.

Dietary Strategies

Navigating menopause requires a thoughtful diet that supports overall health while accommodating the body's changing needs. Practical dietary strategies and meal planning tips are invaluable in this journey, ensuring that each meal contributes to a woman's well-being. Incorporating nutrient-dense foods into daily meals can help address hormonal fluctuations and mitigate menopausal symptoms. Focusing on fruits, vegetables, lean proteins, and whole grains ensures a rich intake of vitamins, minerals, and fiber, promoting digestive health and satiety.

Meal planning during menopause should also prioritize foods rich in phytoestrogens, such as soy products, flaxseeds, and certain beans, which may offer natural hormone balance support. Regular meals help manage metabolic changes and maintain energy levels throughout the day. Additionally, reducing the intake of processed foods, sugars, and excessive caffeine can further align with the body's needs during this transition.

Incorporating these strategies into meal planning not only supports hormonal and physical health but also empowers women to navigate menopause with confidence, ensuring that diet remains a cornerstone of their health strategy.

Combating Weight Gain and Restoring Energy Levels

Understanding Weight Gain

Menopause marks a pivotal time in a woman's life, bringing about significant changes that extend to body composition, including a tendency toward weight gain. This shift is primarily attributed to hormonal changes, particularly the reduction in estrogen levels, which can affect metabolism and fat distribution and increase abdominal fat. Additionally, aging is accompanied by a decrease in muscle mass, further impacting metabolic rate.

Fasting emerges as a strategic tool in addressing these challenges, offering a method to enhance metabolic flexibility and encourage the body to utilize fat stores for energy. By adopting fasting practices, women can influence their body's energy regulation mechanisms, potentially mitigating the metabolic slowdown associated with menopause. Intermittent fasting, for instance, can improve insulin sensitivity and lead to a more efficient metabolic profile, aiding in managing menopausal weight gain.

Understanding the interplay between menopause, weight gain, and fasting is crucial. It empowers women to make informed choices about their health, using fasting not just as a dietary approach but as a holistic strategy to navigate the physical changes of menopause with grace and resilience.

Energy Restoration

During menopause, the quest for energy restoration becomes more crucial than ever. Embracing fasting, sleep optimization, and physical activity can be a powerful trifecta for enhancing energy levels during this transformative phase. Fasting, particularly when tailored to align with your body's natural rhythms, can significantly improve metabolic efficiency, leading to a more vibrant energy state.

The art of sleep optimization plays a pivotal role in this energetic renaissance. Quality sleep rejuvenates the body and mind, making it a critical component of the menopausal journey. Integrating practices such as maintaining a consistent sleep schedule and creating a restful environment can enhance sleep's restorative power, complementing fasting's benefits.

Physical activity, tailored to your body's needs and preferences, catalyzes energy enhancement. Yoga, walking, or swimming boost cardiovascular health and promote endorphin release, contributing to a heightened sense of vitality.

Incorporating these strategies into daily life during menopause can transform the experience into a period of renewal and energy. By focusing on fasting, optimizing sleep, and engaging in physical activity, you can navigate menopause gracefully, embracing the changes with vitality and strength.

Metabolic rate support

Navigating menopause requires a nuanced approach to maintaining metabolic health, with strategies like resistance training and optimal protein intake taking center stage. As estrogen levels fluctuate and eventually decline, the body's metabolic rate can slow, making these strategies vital for supporting metabolic resilience and vitality.

Resistance training emerges as a cornerstone of this metabolic support system. Engaging in strength-building exercises not only helps counteract the muscle mass loss typically associated with aging but also boosts the metabolic rate. This form of physical activity encourages the body to burn calories more efficiently, even at rest, providing a double-edged sword against menopausal weight gain.

Parallel to the benefits of resistance training, prioritizing protein intake plays a critical role in metabolic health during menopause. High-quality protein sources, such as lean meats, legumes, and dairy, are essential for preserving muscle mass and promoting satiety. Incorporating adequate protein into your diet supports the body's thermogenic processes, further enhancing metabolic function.

Resistance training and mindful protein consumption form a powerful duo for supporting metabolic rate during menopause. By integrating these strategies into your lifestyle, you can empower your body to navigate the metabolic shifts of menopause with strength and vitality, laying the foundation for long-term health and well-being.

Share Your Thoughts, Share the Love

Share the Gift of Transformation

"Kindness is a language which the deaf can hear and the blind can see." - Mark Twain

Did you know? Folks who do kind acts without expecting anything in return tend to be happier, live longer, and even find more joy in their daily lives. And if there's a chance for us to spread a little bit of that magic around, you bet we're going to take it!

So, here's something I'm pondering...

Would you be willing to lend a hand to someone you've never met, without any hopes of a thank you?

Now, who's this mystery person, you might wonder? They're a lot like you. Maybe how you were before you discovered the joy and challenges of fasting. They're on the lookout for a change, eager to learn, and in need of guidance but not quite sure where to start.

Our goal is simple: to make the wonders of fasting known to everyone. Every little thing I do is driven by this goal. But to really make it happen, we need to reach... well, everyone.

This is where your superhero powers come in. Believe it or not, a lot of folks decide on a book based on its cover (and what folks say about it). So, on behalf of a fellow fasting newbie you've never met, I'm reaching out with a request:

Could you share a bit of love by leaving a review for this book?

This act of kindness doesn't cost a dime and takes less than a minute, but it could

forever change another person's journey. Your review might help...

...someone regain their health and confidence.

...a mom find balance in her hectic life.

...a woman seeking to understand her body better.

...an individual transform their approach to wellness.

...a dreamer achieve their health goals.

...bring more joy and health to someone's table.

To spread this kindness and make a real difference, all you need to do is take a quick moment to...

leave a review.

Just scan the QR code or click the link below to share your thoughts

»>Leave Amazon Review Click Here«<

If the thought of helping someone out there warms your heart, then you're exactly who we love having in our community. Welcome aboard! You're one of the shining stars in our sky.

I can't wait to continue supporting you on your journey to achieve better health, more energy, and a balanced life faster than you ever imagined. The next chapters are packed with insights you won't want to miss.

A huge thank you from the deepest part of my heart. Now, let's dive back into our adventure.

Your biggest Fan, Patricia B.

PS - Fun fact: When you offer something valuable to someone, you become more valuable in their eyes. If you've found value in this book and think it could help another, why not spread the love and recommend it to them?

Chapter 5: Intermittent Fasting Variations

Exploring 16/8, 5:2, OMAD, and Beyond

Overview of popular methods

In fasting, several methods stand out for their unique approaches and benefits, particularly resonating with women seeking flexibility and effectiveness. The 16/8, 5:2, and One Meal A Day (OMAD) schedules offer diverse options to align with various lifestyles and goals.

The 16/8 method is distinguished by its simplicity and adaptability, involving 16 hours of fasting followed by an 8-hour eating window. This schedule is particularly appealing for its ease of integration into daily routines, allowing most of the fasting period to occur during sleep. It's conducive to maintaining a social life and family meals, making it a sustainable choice for many women.

The 5:2 approach offers a different rhythm, with five days of normal eating and two days of reduced calorie intake, typically around 500-600 calories. This method is praised for its flexibility and is linked to improved insulin sensitivity and brain health. It allows for a break from the rigidity of daily fasting, providing a balance that can be especially beneficial for those new to fasting or with busy schedules.

OMAD takes fasting to a more intense level, condensing the entire day's nutrition into a single meal. This method can significantly simplify meal planning and reduce the time spent on meals, offering profound clarity and focus alongside potential metabolic benefits. However, it requires careful nutritional planning to ensure that all dietary needs are met in that one meal.

Each of these fasting schedules offers unique advantages, from the 16/8 method's compatibility with daily life to the 5:2 approach's balance and OMAD's simplicity and intensity. By understanding the mechanics and benefits of each, women can make informed choices about which fasting method aligns best with their health goals, lifestyles, and personal preferences.

Personal Experience and Adaptation

Embarking on a fasting journey is akin to embarking on a deeply personal voyage of discovery, inviting you to listen intently to your body and respond to its unique needs and signals. The essence of this journey lies not in the adherence to rigid guidelines but in the art of personal experimentation and adaptation. Each woman's body is a distinct universe, with its cycles, rhythms, and nuances, necessitating a tailored approach to fasting that resonates with her physiological and lifestyle needs.

Finding the most suitable fasting method is not a one-size-fits-all path but a dynamic process of trial, reflection, and adjustment. It encourages a mindful exploration of various fasting schedules, attentiveness to the body's responses, and the willingness to modify practices as life's circumstances evolve. This adaptive approach enhances the effectiveness of fasting in promoting health and well-being. It ensures the practice is sustainable, enjoyable, and aligned with one's evolving health goals and life stages.

In this light, the narrative of fasting transforms into one of empowerment, where each woman becomes the expert on her body, learning from her experiences and crafting a fasting practice that celebrates her unique journey towards health and vitality.

Comparative Analysis

Navigating the different fasting methods can be likened to selecting the right tool for a specific wellness goal. Here's a comparative analysis, structured in bullet points, to provide a clearer view of the pros and cons of the 16/8 method, the 5:2 method, and OMAD (One Meal a Day), each enriched with additional insights:

16/8 Method

Pros:

- Easily integrates into daily routines, allowing for social dinners or lunches.
- Enhances insulin sensitivity, supporting weight management and metabolic health.
- Offers flexibility to adjust eating and fasting windows as needed.
- It may improve mental clarity and focus during fasting periods.

Cons:

- The prolonged fasting window might be challenging for beginners or those with high energy needs.
- May lead to overeating in the 8-hour window if not mindful.
- Requires discipline to avoid snacking late at night.
- Some may experience mid-morning hunger, making concentration on tasks more difficult.

5:2 method

Pros:

- Flexibility with five days of normal eating and only two days of calorie restriction.
- Can lead to significant metabolic health benefits with less frequent fasting.
- Encourages nutrient-dense food choices on low-calorie days.
- May be easier to stick with long-term due to less daily restriction.

Cons:

- Calorie-restricted days can be challenging and lead to significant hunger.
- Planning and preparing low-calorie meals require effort and discipline.
- May affect energy levels and exercise performance on low-calorie days.
- The drastic change in daily calorie intake could lead to mood swings.

OMAD (one meal a day)

Pros:

- Simplifies meal planning and preparation by focusing on one main meal.
- Potentially accelerates weight loss and improves metabolic markers.
- Encourages more mindful eating practices and savoring of the meal.
- Can increase growth hormone levels, beneficial for fat loss and muscle preservation.

Cons:

- May be socially isolating or challenging to maintain in social settings.
- Requires careful planning to ensure nutritional needs are met in one meal.
- Not suitable for those with certain medical conditions or high nutritional needs.
- Risk of overeating or making poor food choices due to extreme hunger.

This structured comparison aims to illuminate the path for women seeking to adopt a fasting method that resonates with their lifestyle, health goals, and personal preferences, ensuring an informed and tailored approach to fasting.

Success stories

The first time I embarked on my fasting journey, I chose the 16/8 method, where I fasted for 16 hours and allowed myself an 8-hour window to eat. This approach was new, but I was determined to give it my all. To complement the fasting, I focused on consuming healthy, nutritious foods during my eating window, ensuring that every meal was balanced and beneficial for my body.

This was about more than just fasting and fostering a holistic approach to health and wellness.

After a week of diligently following the 16/8 method, I introduced another fasting strategy into my routine—the 5:2 method. This involved eating normally five days a week and significantly reducing my calorie intake for the remaining two days. The transition was smoother than I anticipated, and before I even completed the second fasting day of the 5:2 method, I experienced a breakthrough. To my astonishment, I had lost more than 5 pounds. The scale, frustrating for so long, reflected my hard work and dedication. The excitement and sense of achievement were unparalleled; it was a moment of pure delight.

Encouraged by this success, I felt motivated to explore different fasting variations further. Each new method I tried brought challenges and rewards, but my initial success with the 16/8 and 5:2 methods was a robust foundation. It was a testament to the effectiveness of fasting when combined with a mindful approach to eating. This experience wasn't just about weight loss; it was a profound journey towards understanding my body's needs and how best to nurture it. My venture into fasting had started as an experiment, but it quickly evolved into a lifestyle that brought me closer to achieving my health and wellness goals.

Customizing Your Fasting Window for Maximum Benefits

Identifying Your Body's Prime Fasting Times

Embarking on a fasting journey invites an intimate dialogue with your body, a process of listening and responding to subtle cues and signals. Identifying your body's prime fasting and feeding times is an art honed through attentiveness and experimentation, allowing for a fasting schedule that harmonizes with your physiological rhythms. This personalized approach enhances the fasting experience, aligning it with natural energy highs and lows, hunger patterns, and lifestyle demands.

The process begins with observing your body's natural hunger signals throughout the day, noting times of heightened energy and those of fatigue. Many find their energy peaks in the morning, suggesting an earlier feeding window might optimize vitality and focus. Others might notice a surge of energy in the evening, indicating a later feeding window could be more beneficial.

Equally important is recognizing how different fasting windows affect your mood, sleep quality, and overall well-being. Adjustments should be made based on these observations, shifting fasting or feeding windows to align with when you feel most energized, focused, and satisfied.

Through this practice of keen observation and adaptation, you can discover the fasting rhythm that feels most natural and supportive, creating a fasting practice that respects and enhances your body's innate wisdom and capacity for health.

Lifestyle Considerations

Incorporating fasting into the intricate tapestry of daily life requires a thoughtful approach that considers the unique rhythms of your routine, work commitments, and family interactions. The key to a sustainable fasting practice lies in its flexibility and adaptability, ensuring it enhances rather than disrupts your lifestyle. You create a harmonious balance supporting your health goals and responsibilities by aligning fasting schedules with personal and professional obligations.

For instance, if your mornings are packed with meetings or school drop-offs, a fasting window that ends in the morning allows you to engage in these activities with energy and focus, followed by a nourishing meal. Conversely, if evenings are your time for family dinners or social gatherings, adjusting your eating window to close with these events ensures you can partake fully in these meaningful interactions.

The objective is to mold your fasting practice around your life, not vice versa. This approach promotes a sense of ease and sustainability, making fasting a natural part of your routine rather than an added stressor. By listening to your body and observing your lifestyle's demands, you can tailor your fasting schedule to serve you best, fostering a sense of well-being that permeates every aspect of your life.

Trial and Error

Embarking on a fasting journey is akin to crafting a bespoke garment; it requires patience, experimentation, and a willingness to adjust until the fit is right. Encouraging a period of trial and error is crucial in discovering the fasting window that resonates best with your body's needs and your lifestyle. This exploratory phase is not about striving for immediate perfection but about embracing the process of learning and adapting.

You may encounter challenges and surprises as you experiment with different fasting schedules. Some days, you find a 16-hour fast to be effortlessly invigorating, while on others, adjusting to a shorter or longer window may feel more aligned with your body's signals and daily demands. This period of trial and error allows you to listen intently to your body's feedback, understanding its cues for hunger, energy levels, and overall well-being.

The beauty of this approach lies in its empowerment, offering you the autonomy to shape your fasting practice into a personalized tool for health and vitality. By granting yourself the grace to adjust and experiment, you pave the way for a fasting experience that yields the best results and fosters a deep connection with your body's innate wisdom.

Nutritional Planning

Navigating the intricacies of nutritional planning within the fasting frame-work is akin to orchestrating a symphony; each meal must harmonize with your fasting and fitness goals, creating a melody of wellness and vitality. This guidance centers on crafting nutrient-dense meals, ensuring that each eating window is an opportunity to nourish your body with the vitamins, minerals, and macronutrients it craves for optimal health.

In this dance of nourishment, balance is critical. Incorporating a variety of whole foods, rich in colorful vegetables, lean proteins, healthy fats, and whole grains, sets the stage for a well-fueled body and a clear and focused mind. By thoughtfully planning your meals, you empower yourself to support your fasting journey, making each bite a step towards achieving your fitness aspirations. This deliberate approach to nutrition enhances your fasting experience and elevates your overall well-being, leaving you energized and prepared to embrace the challenges and joys of life.

The Role of Exercise in Intermittent Fasting

Exercise Timing

In the symphony of fasting and wellness, timing your exercise is like finding the perfect rhythm that complements the melody of your day. The interplay between your fasting and feeding windows offers a unique opportunity to optimize energy levels and recovery, making every workout session more effective and enjoyable. Engaging in physical activity just before your feeding window can amplify the benefits of your post-workout nutrition, allowing your body to absorb and utilize nutrients more efficiently for muscle repair and growth. Conversely, gentle, restorative exercises such as yoga or walking during fasting can enhance fat-burning and mental clarity without depleting your energy reserves. This nuanced approach to scheduling exercise around your fasting and feeding times maximizes your physical performance and aligns your body's natural rhythms with your fitness goals, ensuring a harmonious balance between vigor and recovery.

Type of Exercise

Navigating the landscape of intermittent fasting, women are presented with an exquisite palette of exercise types, each offering unique brushstrokes to the canvas of wellness.

High-Intensity Interval Training (HIIT):

· Boosts metabolism and fat loss with concise, intense sessions.

- Aligns with the fasting ethos of maximizing results efficiently.

Yoga:

- Enhances flexibility and stress reduction with gentle flow and deep breaths.
- Paints a picture of mindfulness and balance during the fasting journey.

Pilates:

- Strengthens the core and improves posture through precision and control.
- Sculpts and tones provide a complementary contour to the fasting form.

These diverse exercise modalities enrich the fasting experience and allow a personalized fitness journey, inviting each woman to find her rhythm and grace in the holistic dance of health and well-being.

Fasting and Muscle Recovery

In the symphony of wellness, intermittent fasting, and muscle recovery compose a harmonious duet. As the body dances through fasting and feeding cycles, understanding the rhythm of muscle recovery becomes paramount. Intermittent fasting, a conductor of metabolic harmony, can influence muscle repair and growth tempo. The key to a harmonious performance lies in the strategic timing of nutrient intake. During feeding windows, a crescendo of protein-rich foods and essential nutrients ensures that muscles receive the building blocks required for repair and growth. This nutritional choreography supports the body's recovery after exercise and enhances the overall benefits of fasting. Embracing this approach allows women to gracefully balance the demands of fasting with the needs of their muscles, ensuring that each step taken on this wellness journey is purposeful and nourishing.

Real-Life Balancing Acts

In the graceful ballet of life, intertwining exercise with intermittent fasting requires finesse and practical wisdom. Drawing inspiration from the real-life experiences of women who've mastered this dance, several helpful tips emerge as guiding stars. First, the art of scheduling exercises during feeding windows, ensuring the body is fueled and ready for movement, transforms workouts into celebrations of strength rather than chores. For those who find dawn's quietude irresistible, a gentle yoga session can harmonize the spirit and body before breaking the fast. Midday walkers, on the other hand, discover the joy of stepping out post-lunch when energy levels peak and nourishment flows through their veins. Evening enthusiasts often reserve strength training for when the day's meals have painted their bodies with energy, allowing for robust sessions that don't deplete but enrich. Each woman's journey weaves her unique pattern, showing that with thoughtful planning and a dash of creativity, fasting and exercise can coexist in beautiful, life-enhancing synergy.

Breaking a Fast: Best Practices for Women

Gentle Reintroduction of Foods

In the tender moments that mark the end of a fast, the reintroduction of foods into one's diet is akin to a gentle whisper, urging the digestive system to awaken from its slumber with grace and ease. This delicate phase calls for a symphony of soft, easily digestible foods that nurture the body and soothe the soul. Beginning with a warm, comforting broth or a light vegetable soup can be a soothing balm for the stomach, gently stimulating digestive enzymes without overwhelming the system. Steamed vegetables, rich in nutrients yet soft on the stomach, follow, introducing fiber in a manner that respects the body's gradual return to its total digestive capacity. Lean proteins and fermented foods, introduced slowly, act as building blocks for recovery and balance, supporting the body's nutritional needs while ensuring digestive harmony. This gentle reawakening of the digestive system, guided by intuition and care, provides that transitioning from fasting to feeding nourishes the body and spirit, making each meal a celebration of renewal and well-being.

Choosing the Right Foods

As the dawn breaks on the completion of a fast, choosing the right foods to grace your plate becomes an art—a delicate dance of flavors and nutrients that replenish and rejuvenate the body with gentle care. The tableau of post-fast nourishment is painted with the vibrant colors of fruits and vegetables; think berries bursting with antioxidants, leafy greens rich in minerals, and avocados full of heart-healthy fats. Each bite is a brushstroke that nourishes the body and delights the senses.

Whole grains like quinoa and brown rice offer a canvas of complex carbohydrates, providing sustained energy and a comforting warmth. Lean proteins, such as grilled salmon or tofu, act as the foundation, rebuilding muscle and supporting cellular repair with their essential amino acids.

Fermented foods, like kefir or sauerkraut, introduce probiotics, whispering life into the gut microbiome, enhancing digestion and absorption of nutrients. These foods, chosen with love and intention, not only replenish the body but also elevate the spirit, transforming eating into a ritual of self-care and gratitude.

Listening to Your Body

In the quiet moments following a fast, the body speaks in whispers and roars, a dialogue of responses to the foods we reintroduce. It is a time of heightened awareness, a sacred opportunity to listen deeply to our bodies' signals. This practice of attentive listening is not just an act of self-care; it's a profound form of self-respect.

As you break your fast, notice how each food resonates with your body. The crunch of an apple, the smoothness of almond butter, or the lightness of a broth—each has its language, telling stories of nourishment, energy, and sometimes, discomfort. Paying attention to these signals—a sense of vitality, a hint of bloating, or an energy dip—guides you toward the foods that truly nourish and rejuvenate your body.

This listening journey is profoundly personal and paved with patience and curiosity. It transforms eating from routine to ritual, inviting a dialogue with your body that enriches your physical well-being and connection to yourself.

Hydration and Supplements

In the tapestry of fasting, hydration and supplements are threads that weave through the fabric of our post-fast nourishment, essential to replenish and revitalize our bodies. As we emerge from the serenity of a fast, our first gesture of kindness is often a sip of water, a simple act that signals to our body the gentle commencement of nourishment. This moment of rehydration is pivotal, as it begins the process of reinvigorating our systems, flushing toxins, and preparing the digestive tract for the foods to come.

Supplements, too, hold a place of honor in this delicate dance of replenishment. Whether it's magnesium to ease relaxation, omega-3s to reduce inflammation, or a B-complex vitamin to boost energy, each supplement is a potential ally selected to support our body's unique needs. Yet, this path is not about mere consumption but a conscious choice, a dialogue between our inner wisdom and the nutrients we invite into our sanctuary.

As we navigate this journey, let us remember that hydration and supplements are not merely acts of filling but of feeling, tuning into our body's rhythm and responding with care. This mindful approach transforms our post-fast nourishment into a practice of self-love, a symphony of actions that resonate with our body's deepest needs.

Chapter 6: Extended and Periodic Fasting

Preparing for Your First Extended Fast

Mental and Physical Preparation

Embarking on an extended fast is akin to setting sail on a profound journey of self-discovery, where preparation is the compass that guides us through the waters of mental and physical readiness. This journey begins not at the dawn of our fasting period but in the nurturing days that precede it, where a clean diet acts as the foundation upon which we build our fasting experience. By leaning into foods that are as close to their natural state as possible—rich in nutrients, low in processed sugars, and abundant in whole grains, fruits, and vegetables—we gently ease our body into a state of readiness, minimizing potential detox symptoms and setting the stage for a smoother transition into fasting.

Setting Realistic Goals and Expectations

Preparing our mind is crucial, a sanctuary that must be cared for. Practices such as meditation, journaling, or simply setting intentions can fortify our mental resilience, creating a space of calm and focus. This holistic approach, balancing both diet and mindfulness, ensures that we step into our fasting journey grounded, prepared, and open to the transformative possibilities that lie ahead.

Venturing into extended fasting is a testament to one's commitment to health and well-being. Yet, setting realistic goals and managing expectations paves the way for success. Embarking on this journey with a clear, attainable objective is a beacon of motivation and a safeguard against the disheartenment that ambitious expectations might sow. For instance, a beginner might aim to complete a 24-hour fast, focusing on the experience rather than immediate, tangible outcomes such as significant weight loss. Another achievable goal is maintaining mindfulness and presence during the fast, observing the body's signals without succumbing to impulsive reactions to hunger.

We foster a sense of achievement and progress by aligning our goals with our current capabilities and gradually expanding our fasting horizons. This approach encourages a sustainable practice, where each fast is a step forward in our health journey, not a leap towards unrealistic ideals. No matter how modest, celebrating these milestones cultivates a resilient fasting mindset emboldened by patience and perseverance.

Safety first

As we navigate the transformative journey of extended fasting, the "Safety First" mantra becomes our guiding principle, illuminating the path toward holistic well-being. This approach underscores the importance of consulting with a healthcare professional before embarking on an extended fast. Such preemptive dialogue is designed to tailor the fasting experience to individual health profiles, ensuring the journey enhances rather than compromises well-being.

The necessity for medical consultation is especially pronounced for those with underlying health conditions such as diabetes, heart disease, or any condition that necessitates regular medication. Women who are pregnant or breastfeeding, as well as individuals with a history of eating disorders, are advised to seek specialized guidance to navigate their fasting journey safely.

Moreover, recognizing the signals that necessitate halting a fast is crucial. Symptoms such as severe dizziness, overwhelming fatigue, acute headaches, or any signs of cognitive impairment indicate that one's body is in distress, warranting an immediate cessation of the fast. These manifestations remind us that the primary goal of fasting is to nourish and fortify our health, not to deplete it. In heeding these signs and consulting with healthcare professionals, we embrace fasting as an act of discipline and profound self-care, ensuring our journey is safe and enriching.

Building Up Gradually

Embarking on the voyage of extended fasting is akin to cultivating a garden; it thrives on patience, care, and the wisdom of gradual cultivation. Just as a seedling is nurtured to bloom, so should one approach the fasting journey, starting with shorter fasts and tenderly extending the duration over time. This systematic progression allows the body to adapt gently to fasting rhythms, fostering a sustainable practice rooted in kindness and attunement to one's physical and mental readiness.

Beginning with intermittent fasting windows, such as the 12/12 or 16/8 method, is the fertile ground from which confidence and comfort with fasting can grow. Over time, as one becomes more attuned to the body's signals and responses, the fasting periods can be carefully extended, perhaps to 24 hours or even to alternate-day fasting, always guided by an ethos of self-respect and mindful observation.

This gradual approach minimizes potential stress on the body and cultivates a deeper connection with the nuances of one's fasting experience. It allows for exploring fasting as a journey of self-discovery, where each step is taken with awareness, and each extension is a testament to one's growing resilience and understanding. In embracing fasting as a practice built gradually, we open ourselves to its transformative potential, ensuring that our journey is practical and imbued with a profound sense of personal achievement and well-being.

Autophagy, Detoxification, and Immune System Reset

Understanding Autophagy

Autophagy, a critical and sophisticated process within the body, is a cornerstone of cellular maintenance and health. This self-degradative system is essential for clearing out dysfunctional or damaged cellular components, ensuring cellular quality control and homeostasis. The term itself, derived from the Greek words "auto," meaning self, and "phagy," meaning eating, aptly describes this process where cells essentially consume and recycle their own parts.

During extended fasting periods, autophagy rates significantly increase. This escalation is due to the body's adaptive response to nutrient scarcity. Without external energy sources, the body shifts its focus internally, identifying and breaking down cellular debris and protein aggregates that can otherwise accumulate and lead to cellular dysfunction. This breakdown process generates amino acids and fatty acids, which are then reused for energy production and the synthesis of new cellular components, demonstrating a remarkable efficiency in resource utilization.

The benefits of autophagy extend beyond mere cellular cleanup. By eliminating potential sources of inflammation and infection, autophagy plays a protective role against many diseases, including neurodegenerative diseases like Alzheimer's and Parkinson's, certain types of cancer, and infections. Furthermore, autophagy contributes to longevity and the delay of aging processes by promoting cellular renewal and preventing the accumulation of damaged cellular components.

The enhancement of autophagy through extended fasting underscores the body's innate wisdom in self-preservation and optimization and highlights the potential of fasting as a therapeutic intervention. Understanding and harnessing this natural process can lead to profound health benefits, making autophagy a critical area of interest in the quest for optimal health and longevity.

Detoxification Processes

Extended fasting acts as a potent trigger for the body's natural detoxification processes, enhancing the body's ability to cleanse and rejuvenate from within, with noticeable benefits extending to improving skin health. This period of food abstention does more than give the digestive system a break; it activates a thorough internal cleansing mechanism that targets accumulated toxins and waste products, including those affecting skin clarity and texture.

As the body turns to its energy reserves during fasting, primarily fat cells, these cells release stored toxins into the bloodstream. These are then processed and eliminated through significant organs, including the liver and kidneys, and crucially for skin health, through the skin itself. This detoxification process can lead to a clearer, more radiant complexion as the body reduces its toxic load, minimizing breakouts and other skin issues associated with toxin accumulation.

Moreover, with the digestive system at rest, the body can redirect its energies towards repair and rejuvenation efforts. This includes enhancing liver function, which is central to detoxification, which benefits skin health by filtering blood and breaking down harmful substances for excretion. Improved liver function optimizes the body's detox pathways, directly reflecting healthier, more vibrant skin.

Fasting also stimulates autophagy, a cellular "cleanup" process that removes damaged components. For the skin, this means a reduction in the accumulation of damaged proteins and other cellular debris, leading to a decrease in inflammation and an improvement in skin elasticity and overall appearance.

In addition, reducing inflammation throughout the body, a direct result of fasting-induced detoxification and autophagy can lead to a noticeable improvement in skin conditions such as acne, eczema, and psoriasis. By supporting the body's natural detoxification systems through extended fasting, individuals can enjoy improved energy levels, immune function, and a significant enhancement in skin health, culminating in a clearer, more youthful complexion that radiates vitality.

Boosting the Immune system

Extended fasting holds the transformative potential to reset and fortify the immune system. This benefit has particular relevance for women navigating the complexities of hormonal fluctuations and life transitions, such as menopause. This period of abstention from food goes beyond mere calorie restriction; it activates a profound physiological shift that can rejuvenate the immune system, making it more efficient and resilient against pathogens and diseases.

Research suggests that extended fasting can reduce inflammation, a root cause of many chronic diseases and a critical factor in immune system dysfunction. By lowering inflammation, fasting helps recalibrate the immune response, potentially reducing the risk of autoimmune conditions, which are notably more prevalent in women.

Moreover, fasting stimulates the production of new white blood cells, the body's critical defender against infections. This renewal process enhances the body's ability to fight off infections and improves its ability to respond to vaccinations, an aspect of particular importance as women age and their immune systems naturally weaken.

Another significant benefit of extended fasting for women is its impact on gut health. The gut is an essential component of the immune system, and fasting can help to improve gut barrier function and modulate the gut microbiome, leading to enhanced immune responses.

Extended fasting also encourages autophagy, a cellular cleanup process that removes damaged and dysfunctional components. This process is crucial for maintaining cellular health and proper immune function. By promoting autophagy, extended fasting helps in the prevention of cellular aging. It supports the body's natural defense mechanisms against diseases, including those that women are statistically more at risk for, such as breast cancer.

Incorporating extended fasting into a health regimen can be a powerful strategy for women seeking to enhance their immune resilience. This practice offers a pathway to improved overall health and empowers women with a proactive approach to aging, hormonal balance, and disease prevention, reinforcing their bodily autonomy and well-being.

Scientific Evidence

In a world where the quest for optimal health spans from the rigor of scientific exploration to the personal stories of those who practice fasting, emerging research offers compelling evidence of the benefits of fasting for women. Studies illuminate how fasting initiates autophagy, a cellular cleanup process crucial for removing damaged cells and generating new ones, thus playing a pivotal role in aging and disease prevention. This self-cleansing mechanism has been linked to improved brain function, enhanced longevity, and a reduced risk of chronic diseases, making it a cornerstone of fasting's health benefits.

Moreover, the detoxification processes activated during fasting periods eliminate toxins and reset the body's metabolic pathways, leading to improved energy levels, better digestion, and, importantly for many women, clearer skin. This natural detoxification supports the liver and kidneys, vital organs in the body's detox pathways, enhancing their ability to function efficiently.

The immune system, too, benefits from fasting. Research indicates that periodic fasting can reset immune system parameters, potentially leading to a more robust defense against infections and diseases. This aspect of fasting is particularly relevant for women, who often experience immune system fluctuations due to hormonal changes.

Scientific studies, such as those published in "Cell Stem Cell" and "The New England Journal of Medicine," provide robust evidence supporting these benefits. They highlight not just the immediate impacts of fasting but also its long-term contributions to health and well-being, making a compelling case for incorporating fasting into a holistic approach to health, especially for women seeking to navigate the challenges of menopause and beyond with grace and vitality.

Reintroducing Foods After Extended Fasts

Strategic Reintroduction Plan

Embarking on a journey through extended fasting is akin to pressing the reset button on your body's intricate systems, particularly for women who navigate the ebb and flow of hormonal changes. As you conclude this transformative experience, a strategic reintroduction plan for foods is paramount to ensure that your body reaps the full spectrum of benefits from your fast. The art of gently awakening your digestive system begins with focusing on easily digestible foods that nourish and prepare the body for more complex meals.

Step one involves hydrating with water or herbal teas, setting a serene stage for digestion. Following this, introduce liquid nutrition, such as homemade bone broths or vegetable soups, rich in minerals and gentle on the stomach. Next, integrate soft foods like cooked vegetables and ripe fruits, which offer fiber and essential nutrients without overwhelming the digestive tract.

For women, notably those mindful of hormonal balance, incorporating foods rich in omega-3 fatty acids, such as flaxseeds and chia seeds, and phytoestrogens, found in fermented soy products, can support the endocrine system post-fast. This gradual, mindful approach optimizes nutrient absorption. It respects the body's adjusted pace, ensuring a smooth transition back to a regular eating pattern while maintaining the clarity, energy, and rejuvenation achieved through fasting.

Listening to Digestive Signals

In the quiet aftermath of an extended fast, your body whispers secrets about its inner workings, primarily through the language of digestion. For women, tuning into these subtle cues can transform post-fast nutrition into a deeply personalized healing process. As you reintroduce foods, listening attentively to your digestive signals is essential, a practice that can illuminate food sensitivities and preferences that go unnoticed.

This attentive listening involves noticing changes in digestion, energy levels, and mood after eating certain foods. For instance, some may discover that dairy, previously a dietary staple, now triggers bloating or discomfort, while others might find renewed vitality in plant-based nutrients. Particularly for women, who may navigate the nuances of hormonal fluctuations, this period can offer insights into how different foods impact hormonal balance, mood, and overall well-being.

Embrace this phase as an opportunity to forge a deeper connection with your body's needs, allowing the feedback from your digestive system to guide you towards foods that truly nourish and support your health post-fast. This personalized dietary awareness enhances digestion and empowers women to make informed choices that support their unique physiological and hormonal landscape.

Nutrient-Dense Foods to Prioritize

As the curtain rises after an extended fast, the stage is set for nutrient-dense superstars to play crucial roles in your recovery and revitalization. For women who nurture life's myriad roles, choosing the right ensemble of foods can be particularly empowering, supporting everything from hormonal balance to bone health.

Begin with a symphony of colorful vegetables and fruits, rich in antioxidants, vitamins, and minerals, to combat oxidative stress and nourish your body deeply. Lean proteins, whether from plant sources like lentils and quinoa or fish rich in omega-3 fatty acids, help repair and build tissues while balancing hormones. Seeds and nuts sprinkled like confetti offer magnesium and healthy fats, which are remarkable for bone density. Pay attention to the power of whole grains and legumes, which provide the complex carbohydrates and fiber essential for sustained energy and digestive health. For women, these foods are not just fuel but functional allies, supporting everything from cardiovascular health to emotional well-being. Prioritizing these nutrient-dense choices post-fast can transform your reintroduction into a rejuvenating journey, aligning your body's needs with the nourishing abundance of nature.

As stated above, the rejuvenating phase post-fast, focusing on specific nutrient-dense foods, can significantly enhance recovery and bolster overall health, particularly for women. Here's a list of ten powerhouse foods, each with its key nutrient and a standout benefit:

- **Spinach**: Rich in Iron and Vitamins A and C. *Benefit*: Supports healthy blood creation and enhances skin health.
- **Salmon**: High in Omega-3 Fatty Acids. *Benefit*: Promotes heart health and aids in reducing inflammation.
- **Almonds**: Packed with Vitamin E and Magnesium. *Benefit*: Boosts brain

health and maintains bone density.

- **Quinoa**: Contains a full spectrum of Amino Acids. *Benefit*: Offers a complete protein source for muscle repair and growth.
- **Blueberries**: Loaded with Antioxidants. *Benefit*: Enhances cognitive function and protects against oxidative stress.
- **Chia Seeds**: Excellent source of Omega-3 Fatty Acids. *Benefit*: Supports cardiovascular health and aids in hydration.
- **Lentils**: Rich in Protein and Fiber. *Benefit*: Promotes digestive health and stabilizes blood sugar levels.
- **Avocado**: High in Healthy Fats and Vitamin K. *Benefit*: Supports heart health and aids in nutrient absorption.
- **Sweet Potatoes**: Packed with Vitamin A and Potassium. *Benefit*: Boosts immune function and supports vision health.
- **Broccoli**: Loaded with Vitamins C and K. *Benefit*: Enhances detoxification processes and supports bone health.

Incorporating these foods into your post-fast meals not only replenishes vital nutrients but also caters to the specific needs of women, supporting hormonal balance, bone density, and overall well-being with every bite.

Avoid Common Mistakes

Breaking an extended fast is a crucial phase that requires careful planning and execution. Here, we highlight some common pitfalls to avoid, ensuring a smooth transition back to your regular diet:

- **Overeating**: Jumping back into large meals can overwhelm your digestive system, leading to discomfort and bloating. Your stomach needs time to readjust to digesting solid foods, so it's essential to start with small, easily digestible meals, and gradually increasing portion sizes is essential.
- **Choosing Processed Foods**: Highly processed foods are often low in nutrients and high in sugar, salt, and unhealthy fats. Consuming these can cause rapid spikes in blood sugar and undo the benefits of fasting. Opt for whole, nutrient-dense foods that provide essential vitamins and

minerals for recovery.

· **Ignoring Hydration**: Failing to hydrate adequately, especially with water and electrolyte-rich drinks, can lead to dehydration. Proper hydration is essential for digestion, nutrient absorption, and overall health, especially after fasting.

· **Skipping Nutrient-Dense Foods**: Remember to include a variety of nutrient-dense foods in your post-fast meals, which can result in nutritional deficiencies. To replenish and nourish your body, incorporate a balanced mix of proteins, healthy fats, and carbohydrates from whole food sources.

· **Rushing the Reintroduction of Foods**: Introducing too many different types of foods too quickly can be hard on your digestive system. Start with simple, non-irritating foods and slowly reintroduce other foods while monitoring how your body reacts.

Avoiding these mistakes ensures a healthier and more comfortable transition back to regular eating, supporting your body's recovery and maintaining the benefits gained from fasting.

Monitoring Your Health: When to Break an Extended Fast

Recognizing Warning Signs

In extended fasting, particularly for women, recognizing when to pause or end a fast is paramount for maintaining health. Our bodies communicate through symptoms and signs, signaling when to reconsider our fasting regimen. Here are key indicators:

· **Extreme Fatigue**: While some tiredness is normal, persistently feeling drained or weak suggests your body may require more nutrients to function correctly.

· **Dizziness and Lightheadedness**: These symptoms can indicate low blood sugar levels or dehydration, necessitating immediate attention to prevent fainting or more severe complications.

· **Irregular Heartbeat**: Experiencing palpitations or an irregular heartbeat is a sign to end your fast, as it may reflect electrolyte imbalances or cardiovascular strain.

· **Severe Mood Swings**: While mood fluctuations are common, extreme irritability, anxiety, or depression during fasting should not be ignored, as these can impact your mental and emotional well-being.

· **Menstrual Irregularities**: Women should be cautious of changes in their menstrual cycle, as fasting can affect hormonal balance. A missed period or significant changes in cycle regularity might require reevaluating fasting practices.

Listening to your body and acknowledging these warning signs is crucial. If any of these symptoms persist, you should end the fast and consult a healthcare professional, ensuring your fasting journey supports your physical and mental health.

Regular Check-Ins

Embarking on an extended fasting journey is a commitment to the fasting process and the practice of regular self-monitoring and professional health evaluations when necessary. For women, these check-ins are crucial to ensure the fasting experience remains beneficial and safe.

Regular self-monitoring involves closely observing your body's reactions to fasting. This includes noting changes in energy levels, mental clarity, and physical signs like hunger or satiety. Recognizing any adverse reactions early and making necessary adjustments to your fasting plan is vital. For women, it's essential to be mindful of any shifts in menstrual cycles or symptoms that could suggest hormonal imbalances, as changes can influence these in diet and routine.

Seeking professional health check-ups before, during, and after an extended fast adds a layer of safety to the process. These consultations can help uncover any underlying conditions that fasting might affect, such as iron deficiency or thyroid issues, which are more common in women. Health professionals can also provide tailored advice based on individual health statuses and fasting objectives.

By integrating these practices into your fasting regimen, you ensure that your journey towards transformation is not only focused on health benefits but also prioritizes your safety and caters to the unique health considerations of women.

Adjusting Fasting Plans

Adapting your fasting strategy to accommodate health feedback and personal experiences is akin to fine-tuning a musical instrument for optimal performance. This practice is especially pertinent for women whose bodies undergo hormonal cycles and changes that can influence their fasting experience and outcomes.

The initial step in adjusting your fasting plan involves keenly listening to your body's signals and responses to fasting. It's about recognizing how different fasting durations, the timing of your eating windows, and the types of foods consumed affect your energy levels, mood, and overall well-being.

Personal experiences, coupled with health feedback—such as changes in weight, blood pressure, or blood sugar levels—serve as invaluable indicators for modifying your fasting regimen. For instance, if you notice increased fatigue or hormonal imbalances, it might be a cue to shorten your fasting periods or adjust your meal composition during eating windows.

For women, it's also essential to consider menstrual cycle phases and potential fertility goals when planning fasting schedules. Adapting your approach might mean aligning more rigorous fasting periods with specific stages of your cycle where energy levels are naturally higher, ensuring that your fasting practice supports rather than detracts from your overall health.

This adaptive strategy champions a personalized approach to fasting that respects and responds to your body's unique rhythms and needs, ensuring a sustainable and enriching fasting journey.

Documenting Your Journey

Embarking on a fasting journey is akin to setting sail on a personal voyage of discovery, where each day brings challenges, triumphs, and insights. For women, documenting this journey can be a powerful tool for tracking progress and reflecting on the profound transformations that occur, both physically and emotionally, over time.

Keeping a journal or diary, whether digital or traditional, allows you to meticulously record your fasting schedules, dietary intake, physical changes, emotional states, and any health improvements you notice. This practice serves as a motivational beacon, guiding you through rough patches, and helps identify patterns or correlations between your fasting regime and various aspects of your health and well-being.

Moreover, documenting your journey creates a personal fasting narrative, offering invaluable insights into what works best for your body. It becomes a testament to your resilience, a source of encouragement, and a personalized fasting blueprint tailored to your unique physiological and emotional landscape.

Chapter 7: Fasting in a Busy World

Fasting on the Go: Tips for Busy Women

Preparation and Planning

In the tapestry of a woman's bustling life, weaving fasting into the daily routine requires art and science, particularly in meal planning and preparation. Success in fasting, especially amidst the whirlwind of work, family, and social commitments, hinges on thoughtful preparation and strategic planning.

Emphasizing the importance of preparing nutrient-dense meals ahead of time cannot be overstated. This foresight ensures you are not reaching for quick, less nutritious options when your feeding window opens due to time constraints or hunger pangs. Instead, you have meals that are both nourishing and satisfying, meticulously chosen to support your body's needs and fasting goals.

Moreover, planning your meals harmonizes your fasting schedule with your lifestyle, seamlessly integrating fasting into your daily life. It transforms fasting from a daunting challenge into a manageable and enjoyable part of your wellness journey, showcasing that with the proper preparation, fasting can indeed fit into even the busiest of schedules.

Quick and Nutritious Meals

In the rhythmic flow of a woman's life, where each day brings challenges and triumphs, finding quick and nutritious meal ideas becomes a cornerstone for successfully integrating fasting into a busy lifestyle. The essence of these meal ideas lies in their simplicity and nutritional density, designed to fit snugly within your eating windows while empowering you with energy and vitality.

Imagine dishes that are as delightful to the palate as they are beneficial to the body—smoothie bowls rich in antioxidants, quinoa salads packed with protein, or vibrant stir-fries teeming with fresh vegetables and lean meats. These meals are quick to prepare and ingeniously designed to support your fasting goals, ensuring that each bite nourishes deeply and sustains you through your fasting hours.

Crafting these meals becomes an act of self-care, a way to honor your body's needs while accommodating the demands of your day. They stand as a testament to that nourishment and convenience coexist, providing the sustenance needed to thrive in fasting and life's constant pace. Some quick recipe ideas to get started are in the appendix.

Hydration Strategies

In the tapestry of fasting, where the body embarks on a journey of renewal and cleansing, hydration emerges as a silken thread, essential for maintaining the harmony and balance of our physical well-being for women navigating the intricacies of fasting amidst the whirlwind of daily commitments, understanding and implementing effective hydration strategies becomes paramount.

Staying hydrated transcends mere water consumption, nurturing the body, ensuring its seamless operation, and enhancing the fasting experience. Envision infuses your day with moments of hydration—sipping on herbal teas that soothe the soul, embracing the freshness of fruit-infused waters, or the simple purity of a glass of water, each serving as a reminder of the body's needs and the care it deserves.

Incorporating hydration into a busy day is an art, one that involves mindful practices like carrying a water bottle as a constant companion or setting gentle reminders that prompt you to pause and drink. Such strategies not only support the physical body during fasting but also serve as self-care that replenishes and rejuvenates the spirit, weaving hydration into the fabric of daily life with grace and ease.

Navigating Social Events and Family Meals

Communication and Compromise

In fasting, particularly for women who balance myriad roles, navigating social meals and events while adhering to fasting protocols becomes a delicate dance. It's a journey that often requires the gentle art of communication and compromise, ensuring that personal health goals harmonize with the social tapestry of family and friends.

Opening dialogues about fasting choices with loved ones transforms into an opportunity to share personal health aspirations and their reasons, fostering understanding and support. It's about crafting a space where individual choices are respected while being flexible and open to adjustments during social gatherings. This might mean planning to align fasting windows with family meals or choosing gatherings that allow for fasting-friendly options.

This approach is about maintaining dietary discipline and nurturing relationships and communal eating experiences for women. It's a testament to the power of open communication, mutual respect, and the shared joy of compromise, weaving fasting into life's social fabric with grace and empathy.

Fasting-Friendly Social Tips

Navigating social events and family gatherings while maintaining fasting commitments presents a unique challenge, especially for women who value their health goals and social connections. The key to harmonizing these aspects lies in adopting fasting-friendly strategies that allow enjoyment and participation without compromising fasting principles.

One practical approach is to focus on what can be consumed during these events. Opting for calorie-free beverages like water, herbal teas, or black coffee can be a practical way to engage in the social fabric of gatherings without breaking your fast. Additionally, carrying a bottle of water can serve as both a hydration source and a subtle way to stay aligned with fasting goals.

Politely declining food offerings is another aspect of navigating social scenarios. A gentle but firm explanation of your current fasting regimen, emphasizing its importance to your health and well-being, can help convey your commitment while expressing gratitude for the offer. This approach maintains your fasting integrity and fosters understanding and respect for your dietary choices in social settings.

Incorporating Fasting into Family Life

Incorporating fasting into family life requires a thoughtful approach that respects individual health goals and the collective dining experience. To introduce fasting concepts to family meals in an inclusive and supportive way, start by involving your family in the planning process. Discuss the benefits of fasting and how it can be integrated into your family's routine without drastically altering shared meal times.

One effective strategy is to align your eating window with the family's main meal of the day, ensuring you can still enjoy quality time together over dinner. For families with varying schedules, consider preparing meals easily adaptable to different eating windows, such as dishes that can be served warm for some members and saved for later for others.

Educating your family on the principles of fasting, emphasizing its health benefits and how it fits into a balanced lifestyle, can foster an environment of support. By making minor adjustments, such as planning and preparing meals that accommodate everyone's needs, fasting can become a harmonious part of family life, promoting health and togetherness.

Managing Peer Pressure

Navigating social settings while maintaining your fasting regimen can sometimes invite questions or pressure from peers curious about your lifestyle choices. Managing peer pressure with confidence and grace begins with owning your fasting journey and recognizing its value. When faced with inquiries or comments, a straightforward yet polite explanation of your fasting approach and its benefits can turn curiosity into respect.

It's important to remember that you're not obligated to justify your personal health choices to anyone. However, sharing your experiences positively and informally can inspire others to consider their health decisions. If you encounter persistent pressure or negativity, gracefully steering the conversation away or suggesting a change in topic can help maintain social harmony.

Your confidence in your fasting journey can empower you and enlighten others, turning potential social challenges into opportunities for advocacy and connection.

Building a Supportive Fasting Community

Finding Like-Minded Individuals

Finding a community of like-minded individuals who share your interest in fasting can be incredibly empowering, especially for women navigating their health and wellness journeys. Engaging with local or online fasting communities offers a space to share experiences, challenges, and successes, providing support and inspiration. These communities can be found through social media groups, health and wellness forums, or local health-oriented events.

For women, these communities often go beyond fasting discussions, touching on topics like balancing fasting with family life, managing hormonal changes, and integrating fasting into a busy lifestyle. Participating in such groups can also lead to friendships and accountability partnerships, which can be invaluable in maintaining motivation and commitment to your fasting goals.

Moreover, these communities can offer a wealth of knowledge from diverse perspectives, including insights into how fasting affects women's bodies differently. Engaging with these groups can enrich your fasting journey with a sense of belonging and shared purpose.

Creating Your Support Network

Crafting a supportive network as you navigate the waters of fasting is akin to weaving a safety net that catches you with understanding, respect, and encouragement. For women whose fasting journeys are often interlaced with unique challenges and triumphs, having friends, family, or colleagues who honor and support their lifestyle choices can be a source of immense strength.

Begin by sharing your reasons for fasting, focusing on the health and wellness benefits that motivate your journey. Educating your circle about fasting's role in your life opens doors to empathy and support. Invite curiosity and questions, offering insights into how fasting aligns with your health goals and lifestyle.

Incorporate fasting into social interactions in ways that feel natural and inclusive. Suggest meeting at places that accommodate your fasting schedule or involve activities not centered around food. Celebrate milestones and share your successes, making your support network a part of your journey.

For women, creating a supportive environment can also mean connecting with others who are fasting, sharing experiences specific to women's health, and fostering a community of mutual encouragement. Whether formed of long-time friends or new allies, this network becomes a pillar of support, enriching your fasting experience with shared understanding and collective empowerment.

Leveraging Social Media for Support

In the digital age, social media emerges as a vibrant oasis of support, inspiration, and community for those exploring fasting, particularly for women seeking to align their wellness journeys with their unique life stages and health needs. Platforms like Instagram, Facebook, and YouTube are teeming with fasting experts, enthusiastic communities, and personal success stories that can illuminate your path, offering guidance, encouragement, and a sense of belonging.

These platforms offer women a unique opportunity to connect with voices that resonate with their experiences—balancing fasting with family responsibilities, managing hormonal changes, or finding fasting-friendly recipes catering to a busy lifestyle. Joining groups or following hashtags like #WomensHealth and #FastingForWomen can lead to discovering tailored advice, motivational stories, and even virtual fasting buddies.

Engage actively by sharing your journey, asking questions, and participating in discussions. This reciprocal exchange deepens your understanding and strengthens the fabric of support, making social media a powerful tool to enhance your fasting journey with the wisdom and camaraderie of a global community.

Sharing Your Story

Every woman's journey in fasting is a tapestry of unique challenges, triumphs, and insights. Sharing your story is not merely an act of self-expression but a beacon of inspiration and support for others navigating similar paths. It fosters a profound sense of community and belonging, reminding us that we are not alone in our quest for health and wellness.

Your narrative has the power to illuminate, encourage, and guide. Whether through social media, blogging, or simply conversing with friends, each shared experience can resonate deeply, offering hope, strategies, and a sense of camaraderie. From overcoming plateaus to discovering the joys of newfound energy, your story can be a lighthouse for someone during their fasting journey.

Embrace the opportunity to contribute to this collective wisdom. By opening up about your fasting adventures, you become an integral part of a supportive network, weaving your strengths and vulnerabilities into a shared tapestry that uplifts and educates. Together, our stories create a vibrant community rich with diverse experiences and bound by a common goal: to live our healthiest, most fulfilled lives.

Balancing Work, Life, and Fasting: Real Women's Stories

Real-Life Challenges and Solutions

Embarking on a fasting journey often intersects with the hustle and bustle of daily life, presenting unique challenges that require creativity and resilience to overcome. The stories of women who have seamlessly woven fasting into their busy schedules are powerful testimonials of determination and adaptability.

One woman, a busy mother of three, found her rhythm by aligning her fasting windows with her children's school hours, ensuring her eating window opened in time for a shared family dinner. Another, a high-powered executive, overcame the temptation of business lunches by advocating for walking meetings, thus staying committed to her fasting goals while fostering a healthier work environment.

A third example comes from a night-shift nurse who adjusted her fasting schedule to match her unconventional work hours, ensuring she could fast during less busy times and eat during breaks. This strategy allowed her to maintain her energy levels and provide the best care to her patients.

Another story involves a freelance writer and entrepreneur who juggles multiple projects. She uses meal prepping during her eating windows to ensure she always has quick, nutritious options that fit her fasting schedule, allowing her to focus on her work without worrying about food.

Each story is a mosaic of strategies, from pre-planning meals to leveraging intermittent fasting apps for reminders and support. These narratives highlight the importance of flexibility, finding what works for you, and the power of community. By sharing their journeys, these women illuminate the path for others, proving that with the right approach, integrating fasting into a busy lifestyle is not only possible but can also be incredibly rewarding.

Workplace Fasting Strategies

Navigating fasting within the contours of a bustling work environment requires both strategic planning and graceful communication, for women balancing the demands of their careers with their commitment to fasting, crafting effective workplace strategies becomes an essential component of their wellness repertoire.

To manage fasting routines at work, consider scheduling lunch meetings as "coffee catch-ups" or walking meetings, allowing you to participate without breaking your fast. For those days packed with back-to-back appointments, keeping hydrating beverages at your desk, such as water, herbal teas, or minimal black coffee, can help you maintain your fasting state while staying refreshed.

When faced with social eating scenarios or team lunches, a polite explanation of your fasting schedule can often lead to understanding and respect from colleagues. Also, you can enjoy a cup of bone broth for lunch, adding needed hydration and electrolytes. This can make you feel like you are still part of lunch. Furthermore, aligning your fasting windows with your work schedule ensures you can enjoy your meals during less hectic parts of the day or once you're home, making your fasting journey seamless with your professional life.

Embracing these strategies not only supports your fasting endeavors but also demonstrates that with a bit of creativity and assertiveness, maintaining a fasting routine in a work setting is feasible and empowering.

Maintaining consistency

In the whirlwind of life's unpredictabilities, maintaining a consistent fasting schedule can seem like navigating through a storm with a compass. For women who often juggle numerous roles and responsibilities, finding that consistency is paramount to their fasting journey's success.

Strategies for maintaining a consistent fasting schedule start with planning and flexibility. Setting a fasting schedule that aligns with your lifestyle and daily routines can create a natural rhythm, making it easier to stick to your plan. Utilize digital tools or planners to track your fasting windows and upcoming events that might require adjustments to your schedule.

Embrace the flexibility to shift your fasting hours as needed without guilt. Life events, such as family gatherings or unexpected work demands, may require you to adapt. Remember, fasting is a journey of self-care, not a rigid set of rules.

Furthermore, establishing a routine around your fasting window, like a morning meditation or an evening walk, can reinforce your commitment. These rituals anchor your day and remind you of your fasting goals, helping to maintain consistency amidst life's ebb and flow.

The Role of Flexibility

Embarking on a fasting journey requires determination and a graceful embrace of flexibility. For women, whose lives are often a tapestry woven with varied threads of work, family, and personal commitments, flexibility in fasting practices isn't just beneficial—it's essential. Recognizing that rigid adherence to fasting windows might not always align with the unpredictable rhythms of daily life, flexibility becomes a cornerstone of a sustainable fasting lifestyle.

Understanding and accepting that some days might necessitate a shorter fasting period or adjusting the timing to fit an impromptu work meeting or family dinner is crucial. This adaptability ensures that fasting enhances your life rather than becoming a source of stress. By prioritizing flexibility, you empower yourself to make fasting a harmonious part of your life, adapting to your body's needs and life's demands with compassion and understanding. This approach fosters a more positive and enduring relationship with fasting, celebrating it as a practice of self-care that molds to your life's unique shape.

Chapter 8: Emotional and Mental Well-being

Fasting and Emotional Health: The Connection

Understanding Emotional Responses to Fasting

Embarking on a fasting journey often unveils a spectrum of emotional responses intricately linked to the physical process of abstaining from food. These responses can be particularly nuanced for women, influenced by hormonal fluctuations and daily stressors. Recognizing and navigating these emotional landscapes is vital to a successful fasting experience.

Common emotional responses to fasting include heightened feelings of irritability, anxiety, or euphoria, reflecting the body's adjustment to a new energy source and the brain's response to changes in blood sugar levels. Strategies for managing these emotions involve mindfulness practices, such as meditation or deep breathing exercises, which can help center your thoughts and calm your mind.

Additionally, maintaining open communication with supportive friends or family can provide an outlet for expressing and processing these emotions. Doing gentle physical activities, like walking or yoga, can also elevate mood and reduce stress.

Understanding that these emotional responses are a natural part of the fasting journey allows for a more compassionate approach to self-care during these times. By employing strategies to manage emotional fluctuations, fasting becomes not just a physical practice but a holistic journey of emotional resilience and growth.

Fasting and Mood Regulation

The intricate dance between fasting and mood regulation presents a fascinating aspect of the fasting journey, particularly for women, whose emotional landscapes may be deeply influenced by physiological changes and daily stresses. Fasting, by its nature, can have a profound impact on mood regulation, offering potential benefits that extend into the realm of mental health.

As the body adapts to fasting, it undergoes a metabolic switch from glucose to ketones as its primary energy source, a transition that can influence neurological health and mood stabilization. This shift promotes mental clarity and cognitive function and may contribute to a sense of emotional balance and well-being.

Moreover, fasting has been associated with enhancing brain-derived neurotrophic factor (BDNF), a protein that plays a critical role in neuron health, resilience to stress, and mood regulation. Increased levels of BDNF during fasting periods could support mood elevation and protect against depressive symptoms.

Exploring the impact of fasting on mood regulation reveals its potential as a tool for physical and mental health optimization. For women navigating the complexities of emotional well-being, fasting offers a pathway to discover a more balanced and harmonious state of mind.

Navigating Emotional Eating

Navigating the nuanced terrain of emotional eating during a fasting journey requires a keen awareness of the body's signals and the mind's narratives. Particularly for women who may experience intensified emotional eating triggers due to hormonal fluctuations or stress, distinguishing between physical hunger and emotional cravings is a pivotal skill for maintaining fasting discipline and nurturing overall well-being.

One effective strategy involves pausing to assess hunger cues with mindfulness, asking oneself whether the hunger is physical or stems from an emotional need, such as boredom, stress, or sadness. Implementing a "waiting period" before acting on the impulse to eat can help clarify the true nature of hunger.

Journaling can also be a powerful tool, allowing reflection on the emotions and circumstances preceding cravings. This practice can uncover patterns, making it easier to identify emotional eating triggers.

Developing a repertoire of non-food responses to emotional needs, such as taking a walk, practicing deep breathing, or engaging in a hobby, can provide alternative coping pathways.

By employing these strategies, women can navigate the complexities of emotional eating during fasting, fostering a deeper connection to their bodies and emotions and supporting their journey toward health and balance.

Support Systems For Emotional Eating

In the intricate journey of fasting, the tapestry of emotional health is interwoven with the need for a supportive community. For women, navigating the emotional challenges during fasting underscores the importance of cultivating a robust support system. This network, composed of friends, family, or fellow fasting enthusiasts, is a pillar of strength, offering encouragement, understanding, and shared experiences.

Establishing such a support system can begin with open conversations about your fasting journey, inviting those close to you to understand your goals and the emotional hurdles you might face. Joining online forums or local groups dedicated to fasting provides an opportunity to connect with others on similar paths, fostering a sense of belonging and mutual support.

Additionally, professional guidance from healthcare providers or counselors specializing in nutritional well-being can offer invaluable support, providing tailored advice and coping strategies.

A support system acts as a safety net, ensuring that when emotional challenges arise, you're not alone. This collective strength bolsters your fasting journey and enriches your emotional resilience, illuminating the path to wellness with the warmth of shared support and understanding.

Coping Strategies for Stress and Emotional Eating

Identifying Stress Triggers

For women embarking on a fasting journey, intertwining stress with daily life can present unique challenges, particularly influencing fasting practices and leading to emotional eating. Identifying personal stress triggers is critical to navigating these challenges gracefully and resiliently.

Everyday stress triggers include work deadlines, family responsibilities, or personal relationships, each capable of prompting a turn towards food for comfort. Hormonal fluctuations throughout the menstrual cycle can also heighten stress responses, further complicating the relationship between stress and eating behaviors.

Solutions to these triggers lie in cultivating mindfulness and stress-reduction techniques. Practices such as meditation, yoga, or even short, daily walks can significantly lower stress levels, creating a more conducive environment for successful fasting. Additionally, keeping a journal can help track patterns in stress-related eating, providing insights into how best to manage these moments.

For moments when stress feels overwhelming, turning to a support network for encouragement or distraction can be incredibly effective. Whether through conversation with friends or participation in a fasting community, sharing experiences can lighten the emotional load, making it easier to stay aligned with fasting goals and resist stress-induced eating temptations.

Stress Management Techniques

Managing stress becomes beneficial and essential in the delicate balance of fasting and daily life. For women, integrating stress management techniques into their fasting regimen can enhance the fasting experience, providing a holistic approach to wellness that nurtures both body and mind. Exercise is a powerful ally, releasing endorphins that naturally elevate mood and alleviate stress. Physical activity can be tailored to fit your fasting schedule, whether a brisk walk, a yoga session, or a more vigorous workout. It offers a dual benefit of stress relief and physical health.

Journaling, too, offers a reflective escape, allowing for the processing of thoughts and emotions that might otherwise fuel stress. Setting aside time to write will enable you to create a space for self-expression and clarity, which can be particularly therapeutic during fasting.

Deep breathing exercises serve as a quick and effective tool for immediate stress relief, accessible at any moment of the day. Techniques such as the 4-7-8 method or box breathing can be practiced almost anywhere, providing a simple yet profound way to calm the mind and reduce stress.

Incorporating these stress management techniques into your fasting journey helps you navigate emotional challenges and enriches your overall well-being, making fasting more enjoyable and sustainable.

Mindful Eating Practices

Within the rhythmic flow of fasting and feasting, mindful eating emerges as a harmonious practice, especially for women seeking to deepen their connection with food and honor their bodies. This conscious approach to eating encourages entire presence during meals, allowing for a profound appreciation of flavors, textures, and the nourishing qualities of food. By engaging all senses, mindful eating transforms each meal into a meditative experience, fostering a sense of gratitude and satisfaction.

For women, this practice holds particular significance, as it prevents overeating by enhancing cues of fullness and satisfaction and serves as a gentle reminder of self-care and the importance of nourishing oneself with intention. Mindful eating during eating windows can also be an empowering act of reclaiming one's relationship with food, moving away from cycles of restriction and indulgence to a place of balance and joy.

Incorporating mindful eating practices into your fasting regimen invites a deeper understanding of your body's needs, preferences, and responses to food, enriching the fasting journey with insights and a renewed sense of well-being.

Seeking Professional Support

In the nuanced journey of fasting, recognizing when to seek professional support for emotional eating or stress management is pivotal to nurturing your overall well-being. Understanding the signs that indicate a need for professional guidance is crucial for women, who may navigate complex emotional landscapes influenced by hormonal fluctuations, life transitions, and societal pressures.

When fasting becomes intertwined with emotional eating patterns or when stress seems insurmountable despite self-managed techniques, it may be time to reach out for support. Signs to watch for include consistent overeating during feeding windows, fasting motivated by emotional distress rather than health, or stress impacting daily functioning.

Seeking professional help can begin with a conversation with your health-care provider, who can offer referrals to nutritionists, therapists, or counselors specialized in eating disorders and stress management. These professionals can provide tailored strategies and support, offering a compassionate space to explore the root causes of emotional eating and stress and develop personalized coping mechanisms.

Embracing professional support as part of your fasting journey signifies a commitment to holistic health, acknowledging that wellness often requires a collective mind, body, and spirit effort.

The Psychological Benefits of Fasting for Women

Enhanced mental clarity

Fasting unfolds as a journey of physical transformation and mental rejuvenation, offering a pathway to enhanced clarity and focus. For women, this aspect of fasting can be particularly empowering, illuminating their personal and professional landscapes with newfound clarity and concentration. The metabolic shift during fasting, where the body transitions from glucose to ketones as its primary energy source, plays a pivotal role in this mental enhancement. Ketones, lauded for their neuroprotective benefits, fuel the brain more efficiently than glucose, leading to improved cognitive functions, including sharper focus, better memory retention, and heightened problem-solving abilities.

This enhanced mental clarity opens doors to personal growth and professional advancement, enabling women to tackle challenges with greater ease and confidence. Whether it's pursuing creative endeavors, making strategic decisions, or simply managing daily tasks with more agility, the mental benefits of fasting support women in achieving their goals with a clear mind and a strong sense of purpose. Embracing fasting as a holistic practice thus not only nurtures the body but also cultivates a vibrant, focused mind, laying the foundation for continued growth and success.

Increased Self-discipline and Control

Fasting, in its essence, is a practice of introspection and restraint, offering a unique opportunity to cultivate greater self-discipline and control, particularly in the realm of food choices and eating habits. For women, this discipline extends beyond the table, weaving into the fabric of their daily lives, empowering them with the strength to make mindful decisions.

The act of fasting sets the stage for a deeper understanding of hunger cues and the distinction between physical hunger and emotional cravings. This awareness fosters a heightened sense of control, enabling women to navigate their dietary choices with intention and wisdom. As fasting periods encourage reflection on the reasons behind food consumption, they naturally lead to more disciplined eating patterns, choosing nourishment that genuinely benefits the body and soul.

This journey of self-discipline through fasting not only reshapes one's relationship with food but also instills a sense of mastery that permeates other areas of life. It's a testament to the power of fasting to transform not just the body but also the mind, equipping women with the resilience and determination to pursue their goals with confidence and clarity.

Positive Self-image and Confidence

Fasting, with its deep roots in transformation and renewal, offers more than just physical health benefits; it is a catalyst for fostering a positive self-image and bolstering confidence among women. As they navigate the challenges and triumphs of their fasting journeys, achieving health goals affirms their strength, discipline, and dedication.

Setting, pursuing, and reaching health milestones through fasting instills a profound sense of accomplishment and self-respect. Each fasting cycle completed, each craving resisted, and each health milestone achieved contributes to a growing sense of self-efficacy and body positivity. Women begin to view their bodies not as projects to be fixed but as vessels of strength and capability deserving of care and respect.

Moreover, the mental clarity and emotional balance often accompanying fasting further enhance this positive self-image, empowering women to carry themselves confidently in their personal and professional lives. This newfound confidence, rooted in the discipline and self-awareness developed through fasting, radiates outward, influencing all facets of life and inspiring others.

Connecting with Your Inner Self

Fasting serves as a gateway to deeper self-exploration, offering quiet moments away from the daily feast of life to connect with one's inner self. For women, these periods of fasting become sacred spaces for introspection, where the noise of external demands dims, allowing the inner voice to emerge more clearly. This practice of deliberate pausing nurtures the body and cultivates a fertile ground for personal reflection and growth.

Fasting encourages mindfulness that can illuminate personal desires, fears, and dreams, offering insights that might remain obscured in the hustle of nourished routines. In this reflective state, women can reevaluate their life's priorities, goals, and the alignment between their actions and their deepest values.

This connection to the inner self strengthens resilience, self-awareness, and a profound sense of purpose. Fasting becomes not just a physical discipline but a spiritual journey, enriching the tapestry of life with greater clarity, peace, and personal fulfillment.

Fasting as Self-Care: Mindfulness and Meditation Practices

Integrating Mindfulness

Integrating mindfulness into fasting routines elevates the experience from a mere dietary practice to a holistic self-care journey for women. This fusion of mindfulness with fasting transforms each fast moment into an opportunity for deeper self-connection and presence, enriching the fasting journey with layers of awareness and gratitude.

To weave mindfulness into fasting, begin with intentional meal times during your eating windows. Approach each meal with gratitude, fully engaging with the flavors, textures, and nourishment your food provides. During fasting periods, use the time you might have spent on meal preparation and eating to engage in mindful practices such as meditation, deep breathing exercises, or gentle yoga. These practices not only fill the space with peace and reflection but also help manage hunger and focus on the body's internal cues.

Additionally, journaling before breaking your fast can offer insights into your emotional state and hunger levels, fostering a conscious reconnection with your eating habits. Integrating mindfulness into your fasting routine transforms it into a nurturing space for growth, self-discovery, and enhanced well-being, making each fasting day closer to holistic health.

Meditation and Fasting

Meditation and fasting share a symbiotic relationship, each enhancing the other in the pursuit of mental and emotional well-being. For women, this combination offers a powerful toolkit for navigating the complexities of life with grace and resilience. With its roots in mindfulness and self-awareness, meditation serves as a perfect companion to fasting, deepening the reflective quality of the fasting journey.

Meditation during fasting can amplify the clarity and tranquility that fasting induces. It provides a structured opportunity to quiet the mind, reduce stress, and cultivate inner peace. This mental stillness can make the physical aspects of fasting more manageable, transforming potential moments of hunger or discomfort into opportunities for growth and reflection.

Furthermore, meditation can enhance the emotional resilience that fasting develops, offering strategies to manage cravings and fluctuations and the emotional challenges that may arise. For women, integrating meditation into fasting routines supports their physical health goals. It fosters emotional balance, self-compassion, and a profound connection to their inner selves, enriching their well-being.

Self-Care Rituals

During the sacred windows of fasting, embracing self-care rituals becomes a nurturing embrace for both body and mind, particularly for women who are often the nurturers themselves. These practices can transform fasting periods into times of deep self-renewal and connection.

Consider gentle yoga or stretching to stay engaged with your body, honoring its strength and flexibility without the demand for intense energy expenditure. Engaging in a skincare routine or a warm bath can serve as a reminder of the beauty of self-care, offering a sense of luxury and tranquility.

Mindful walks in nature provide a dual benefit of light exercise and the calming influence of the natural world, while creative outlets like journaling, painting, or knitting allow for expression and mindfulness. Practicing gratitude through reflection or writing can elevate the fasting experience, fostering a positive mindset and deeper appreciation for the journey.

Incorporating these self-care rituals into fasting windows nurtures the body and mind. It enhances the fasting experience, making it a holistic practice of wellness and self-love, specially tailored for women.

The Holistic Approach

Embracing fasting within the broader spectrum of a holistic approach to health invites a transformation that transcends mere dietary discipline, weaving together the physical, mental, and emotional threads of well-being. This comprehensive perspective is beneficial and essential for women, recognizing that proper health flourishes only when all aspects of the self are nurtured in harmony.

Viewing fasting as one element of this holistic tapestry encourages a deeper engagement with the practice, where its physical benefits are celebrated alongside its capacity to foster mental clarity, emotional resilience, and spiritual growth. Incorporating mindful practices, such as meditation and yoga, enhances the mental and emotional dimensions of fasting, turning it into a period of introspection and renewal.

Nutrition also plays a critical role in this holistic model, focusing on nourishing the body with whole, nutrient-dense foods during eating windows to support fasting. By acknowledging and addressing the interconnectedness of the physical, mental, and emotional aspects, fasting becomes a profound journey of self-discovery and holistic health, offering women a path to a balanced and enriched life.

Chapter 9: Building Your Fasting Lifestyle

Beyond the Fast: Creating a Life That Supports Fasting

Holistic Health approach
Adopting a holistic health approach means recognizing fasting as a vital component within a larger constellation of well-being practices. This perspective invites an exploration beyond the physical dimensions of fasting, integrating it with mental, emotional, and spiritual health strategies to cultivate a fully rounded sense of well-being. For women, this holistic approach underscores the importance of nurturing every facet of health, acknowledging the interconnectedness of our bodily systems and the impact of our emotional and mental states on our overall health.

Incorporating fasting into this comprehensive model involves pairing it with other health-promoting practices such as balanced nutrition, regular physical activity, adequate rest, and stress management techniques. This ensures that fasting is not an isolated practice but part of a synergistic regimen that supports and enhances overall health.

By embracing fasting within the broader context of holistic health, it becomes a powerful tool for self-care, offering women a pathway to physical health, mental clarity, emotional balance, and spiritual growth, contributing to a more prosperous, more vibrant life.

Lifestyle Synergy

Creating a lifestyle synergy, where fasting practices harmonize with other lifestyle choices, amplifies the benefits and enriches the overall journey toward well-being. For women, integrating fasting with complementary lifestyle habits can enhance physical health, mental clarity, and emotional stability, crafting a holistic approach to living that supports and sustains their well-being.

To achieve this synergy, consider coupling your fasting routine with a balanced, nutrient-dense diet during eating windows. Opt for whole foods, rich in vitamins, minerals, and antioxidants, to nourish your body and support the detoxification and healing processes that fasting initiates.

Physical activity, tailored to your energy levels and fasting schedule, can also play a crucial role. Gentle yoga or walking during fasting periods can maintain energy and focus, while more intense exercises like strength training or cardio can be scheduled for feeding times to leverage the fuel provided by meals.

Mindfulness practices, such as meditation or deep-breathing exercises, complement fasting by enhancing mental clarity and emotional resilience. Similarly, ensuring quality sleep each night supports the body's regenerative processes, making fasting a more effective and rejuvenating experience.

By aligning fasting with these critical lifestyle choices—nutrition, exercise, mindfulness, and rest—women can create a powerful synergy that fosters physical health and a vibrant, holistic sense of well-being.

Continuous Learning

Embarking on a fasting journey is akin to a lifelong journey of discovery and growth, where continuous learning becomes the compass guiding your path. For women, delving deeper into nutrition, wellness, and fasting is not just about gathering information but refining and enhancing their fasting practice, ensuring it evolves with their changing needs and aspirations.

Encouraging ongoing education allows exploring the latest research, emerging trends, and holistic health strategies that can inform and inspire your fasting routine. Whether it's understanding the science behind autophagy, exploring the benefits of plant-based nutrition, or learning new mindfulness techniques to support your fasting journey, each piece of knowledge adds depth and dimension to your practice.

Attending workshops, reading books, participating in webinars, or joining fasting communities can all be valuable resources for continuous learning. This commitment to education empowers women to make informed decisions about their health, adapt their fasting practices as needed, and navigate their wellness journeys with confidence and curiosity, fostering an effective, enriching, and fulfilling practice.

Case Studies

The tapestry of fasting is rich with stories of transformation and balance, where individuals from diverse backgrounds have successfully integrated fasting into their health-oriented lifestyles. These case studies serve as beacons of inspiration, illustrating the profound impact that mindful fasting can have on overall well-being.

One such story comes from a woman in her mid-forties who embraced intermittent fasting after years of struggling with weight fluctuations and energy levels. Coupling her fasting regimen with a plant-based diet and regular yoga practice, she witnessed a remarkable shift in her health, reporting a significant weight loss and an increase in vitality and mental clarity.

Another example features a busy executive who found fasting the key to managing her stress and improving her focus. By adopting a 16/8 fasting schedule and prioritizing whole, nutrient-dense foods during her eating windows, she navigated her demanding career with renewed energy and resilience, showcasing the power of fasting to support both physical and mental health.

These stories, and countless others like them, highlight the versatility of fasting as a practice that can be tailored to fit each individual's unique needs and goals. They underscore the potential of fasting to be a cornerstone of a balanced, health-oriented lifestyle, providing a source of motivation and a roadmap for those looking to embark on their fasting journey.

The Role of Community in Sustaining Fasting Practices

Finding Your Tribe

In the fasting journey, finding your tribe—a community or group that shares your interests and goals—can be as nourishing for the soul as fasting is for the body. For women, this connection holds particular significance, offering a space of understanding, encouragement, and shared experiences that can significantly enhance the fasting journey.

A supportive community provides more than just companionship; it offers a wealth of collective wisdom, motivation during challenging times, and celebration of milestones achieved. Whether through online forums, social media groups, or local meet-ups, engaging with others navigating similar paths can illuminate your journey, providing insights and strategies that might not have been discovered alone.

This sense of belonging to a fasting tribe encourages accountability, fosters deeper engagement with the practice, and reinforces the commitment to health and wellness goals. This connection can be particularly empowering for women, creating a supportive network that understands the unique challenges and triumphs of fasting from a female perspective.

Finding your tribe is integral to the holistic fasting experience, enriching the journey with camaraderie and shared purpose and reminding us that while fasting may be practiced individually, the journey can be profoundly communal.

Community Resources

In the vast landscape of fasting, navigating the myriad available resources can significantly enhance your journey, connecting you with like-minded individuals and communities dedicated to the practice. Engaging with these resources offers invaluable support, education, and camaraderie for women, making the fasting experience both enriching and more manageable.

Local meetups provide a sense of community and offer opportunities to share experiences, tips, and challenges. These gatherings can range from educational seminars to casual coffee chats, all centered around fasting and wellness.

Online forums and social media groups are treasure troves of information and support, accessible from anywhere. Platforms like Reddit, Facebook, and specialized health websites host vibrant communities where fasting enthusiasts can exchange advice, success stories, and scientific insights. These digital spaces also often include discussions tailored to women's fasting experiences, addressing specific concerns such as hormonal balance, menstrual cycles, and integrating fasting with family life.

Engaging with these community resources broadens your understanding of fasting and provides a supportive network that inspires and sustains your commitment to health. Whether through local meetups or online forums, connecting with others on this journey reinforces the idea that fasting is not just a solitary endeavor but a shared path to wellness.

Collective Wisdom

Tapping into the collective wisdom of the fasting community offers a well-spring of knowledge, inspiration, and support, invaluable for navigating the ebb and flow of the fasting journey. This communal reservoir of experiences becomes a powerful tool for overcoming challenges and bolstering motivation, especially for women who may encounter unique obstacles.

Leveraging the insights and strategies shared by others who have traversed similar terrain allows for a richer, more informed approach to fasting. A sense of solidarity is forged in the shared stories of triumph over cravings, the tips for managing social gatherings, and the advice for aligning fasting with the menstrual cycle. This collective wisdom illuminates the way, offering practical solutions and emotional support that can turn hurdles into stepping stones.

Engaging with the community through forums, social media, or group meetings enhances personal knowledge and contributes to the communal pool of wisdom. It's a reciprocal exchange where every question answered and every experience shared enriches the collective understanding, keeping the flame of motivation alight for all and showcasing the strength of unity.

Giving Back

In the communal fasting journey, giving back by sharing your knowledge and experiences enriches the collective pool of wisdom. It fortifies the bonds within the fasting community for women who often navigate their fasting paths with unique insights and challenges. Contributing their stories and strategies can be a powerful way to support and uplift others embarking on similar journeys.

Encouraging readers to share their successes, lessons learned, and even the hurdles they've overcome invites them to participate in a larger conversation that thrives on mutual support and shared growth. Whether through online forums, social media platforms, or local support groups, each contribution helps to demystify fasting, making it more accessible and less daunting for newcomers.

By giving back, you provide encouragement and guidance to others and reinforce your understanding and commitment to fasting. This cycle of support and sharing fosters a vibrant, nurturing community where every member, from the novice to the seasoned faster, benefits from the collective wisdom and camaraderie, making the fasting journey a shared adventure towards health and well-being.

Fasting and the Planet: Ethical Eating Considerations

Sustainability and Fasting

Fasting, with its roots deeply embedded in the practice of intentional abstention, naturally paves the way for more sustainable and ethical eating habits. This mindful approach to consumption invites individuals, especially women, to reevaluate their relationship with food, fostering a deeper appreciation for the resources that nourish us.

By incorporating fasting into their lifestyle, many shift towards choosing quality over quantity, gravitating towards whole, nutrient-dense foods that support their health goals and have a lesser environmental impact. The practice encourages reducing food waste, as focusing on eating windows leads to more thoughtful meal planning and preparation, ensuring that each bite is purposeful and nourishing.

Furthermore, fasting can inspire a move towards local and seasonal eating, connecting individuals with their communities and the earth's natural cycles. This alignment with the rhythms of nature enhances personal well-being and contributes to a more sustainable and ethical food system.

In embracing fasting, we find a pathway to personal health and a deeper engagement with the world around us, promoting eating habits that are in harmony with the planet and its inhabitants and fostering a more mindful, sustainable approach to our daily nourishment.

Mindful Consumption

Embracing mindful consumption within the fasting framework extends beyond personal health, touching the broader canvas of environmental stewardship and ethical living. This conscious approach to eating encourages a deep consideration of food sources, waste reduction, and the ecological footprint left by our dietary choices. For women, integrating mindfulness into their fasting and eating practices offers a powerful means to connect with and contribute positively to the world around them.

Individuals can support sustainable farming practices and reduce the environmental toll of long-distance food transportation by choosing locally sourced, organically grown, and seasonally appropriate foods. Mindful consumption also involves being aware of packaging and opting for products that minimize plastic use and food waste, aligning with a more eco-friendly lifestyle.

Furthermore, considering the environmental impact of dietary choices, such as the high resource usage of meat production, can lead to a more plant-centric diet, which is healthful and kinder to the planet. Encouraging mindfulness during fasting becomes a vehicle for personal transformation and fostering a healthier, more sustainable world.

Plant-based Fasting

Combining fasting with a plant-based diet is a synergistic approach that amplifies health benefits while honoring environmental stewardship. For women, this alignment offers a holistic pathway to wellness, nurturing the body with nutrient-rich, plant-based foods during eating windows and leveraging the cleansing and restorative powers of fasting.

Adopting a plant-based diet during fasting supports cardiovascular health and weight management. It reduces inflammation thanks to the high intake of antioxidants, fibers, and phytonutrients in fruits, vegetables, legumes, and whole grains. This dietary pattern enhances the detoxification processes that fasting initiates, providing the body with the optimal fuel to repair and rejuvenate.

From an environmental perspective, a plant-based diet requires fewer resources to produce, reduces greenhouse gas emissions, and minimizes water usage, making it a compassionate choice for the planet. By intertwining fasting with plant-based eating, women can forge a path that elevates their health and contributes positively to the world, embodying an ethos of care that extends beyond the self to the global community.

Grass-fed Meats are also Sustainable

Incorporating grass-fed meats into a fasting regimen presents a thoughtful fusion of health optimization and environmental consciousness. Turning to grass-fed meats offers a compelling path for women seeking to align their fasting practices with sustainable and ethical food choices. These meats, sourced from animals raised on natural pastures rather than through conventional, commercial means, stand out for their nutritional, environmental, and ethical advantages.

Grass-fed meats are richer in essential nutrients beneficial for health, including higher levels of omega-3 fatty acids, antioxidants, and conjugated linoleic acid, all of which contribute to reduced inflammation, enhanced heart health, and improved body composition. This nutritional profile complements the health goals of fasting, making grass-fed meats a supportive choice for eating windows.

Environmentally, grass-fed animal farming practices are more sustainable than conventional methods, promoting healthier soils, better water conservation, and reduced greenhouse gas emissions. This approach to animal husbandry aligns with the principles of regenerative agriculture, supporting biodiversity and ecosystem health.

Women can enrich their fasting journey by choosing grass-fed meats with high-quality proteins that support their health goals and contribute to a more sustainable and ethical food system. This choice reflects a commitment to personal well-being and the planet's health, embodying a holistic approach to fasting and nutrition.

Global Movements

Around the globe, a confluence of initiatives and movements is weaving fasting practices with sustainability and ethical consumption, heralding a transformative approach to health and environmental stewardship. These movements, diverse in their reach and focus, share a common vision: to promote dietary choices that benefit individual well-being and the planet's health.

One such initiative is the advocacy for Meatless Mondays. It encourages individuals to embrace plant-based meals at the start of the week, aligning with fasting principles to reduce meat consumption and its associated environmental impact. Similarly, the Slow Food movement emphasizes local, organic eating practices that complement fasting by encouraging mindfulness about food origins and consumption impact, fostering a deeper connection with food.

Global fasting challenges, often organized around environmental events like Earth Day, invite participants to fast as a form of solidarity with those affected by food scarcity, highlighting the power of collective action in addressing global issues.

These movements illuminate the potential of integrating fasting with sustainability and ethical consumption, showcasing how personal health practices can ripple outward, contributing to a more conscientious and sustainable world.

Embracing Change: Your Evolving Fasting Journey

Adapting to Life's Changes

Much like life's journey, Fasting is not a static practice but one that flows and evolves in harmony with the undulating rhythms of health, age, and circumstances. Acknowledging and embracing the need for this evolution in fasting practices is crucial, especially for women, as their bodies navigate through the myriad stages of life, each with its unique demands and shifts.

As health conditions emerge or change, fasting routines may require adjustments to accommodate new dietary needs or medical advice. Similarly, as women age, metabolic rates, and nutritional requirements transform, necessitating a reevaluation of fasting schedules and eating windows to align with these changes.

Life's circumstances, too, play a pivotal role in shaping fasting practices. Major life events, shifts in work schedules, or changes in family dynamics can all prompt a reassessment of how fasting fits into the broader picture of daily life.

Embracing the fluidity of fasting practices in response to these changes is a testament to the resilience and adaptability of the human spirit. It underscores the importance of listening to one's body and being open to modification, ensuring that fasting remains a nourishing and supportive pillar in life's ever-changing landscape.

Personal Growth

Embarking on a fasting journey transcends the mere act of abstaining from food; it unfolds as a profound pathway to personal growth, self-discovery, and an enriched self-care practice. This journey offers women a unique lens to explore their inner landscapes, uncover strengths, confront vulnerabilities, and cultivate a deeper self-awareness.

Fasting challenges individuals to confront their habitual patterns of eating, thinking, and responding to their bodies' cues, inviting a transformative process of learning and adaptation. This introspective voyage can reveal insights about one's relationship with food, body image, and emotional well-being, opening doors to healing and self-acceptance.

Moreover, the discipline and resilience developed through fasting extend beyond dietary habits, influencing broader aspects of life. The practice nurtures patience, perseverance, and mindfulness, which foster a life of intention and purpose.

Viewing fasting as a journey of personal growth enriches the experience, making it not just a quest for physical health but a holistic adventure towards a more conscious, centered, and caring existence. This perspective empowers women to embrace fasting as an act of self-love, a commitment to their well-being, and a celebration of their unfolding journey of self-discovery.

Resilience and Flexibility

Cultivating resilience and flexibility in fasting and health is akin to nurturing a garden through the changing seasons; it requires adaptability, patience, and a deep understanding of the cyclical nature of growth. For women, embracing this approach to fasting and overall well-being is especially poignant, reflecting the ebb and flow of their unique physiological and life experiences.

Resilience in fasting is about more than enduring hunger; it's about embracing each challenge as an opportunity for learning and strengthening one's commitment to health. It involves recognizing that setbacks or deviations from the fasting plan are not failures but part of the journey, offering valuable insights for adjustment and growth.

Flexibility is equally vital, allowing for the modification of fasting routines to align with the body's changing needs, whether due to menstrual cycles, life stressors, or health conditions. This adaptable approach ensures that fasting remains a supportive practice, enhancing well-being without becoming a source of additional stress.

By fostering resilience and flexibility, women can gracefully navigate their fasting and health journey, embracing each phase with confidence and self-compassion and recognizing the beauty in their capacity to adapt and thrive amidst life's constant changes.

Legacy of Health

Embarking on a fasting journey is not just a personal quest for health and well-being; it's an opportunity to contribute to a legacy of wellness that transcends individual experience. For women, this perspective offers a powerful motivation to embrace fasting as a tool for personal transformation and a gift of knowledge and inspiration they can share with others.

This legacy of health is built on the foundations of self-care, resilience, and empowerment gained through fasting. It's about more than the physical benefits; it's the lessons learned, the mental clarity achieved, and the emotional balance nurtured. By sharing these experiences with family, friends, and community, women can inspire and support others in their health journeys, creating ripples of positive change.

Viewing fasting as part of a broader legacy encourages a deeper engagement with the practice, making it a meaningful aspect of life's work. It transforms fasting into a contribution to collective well-being, a beacon of health and wellness that lights the way for future generations, embodying the power of shared knowledge and the strength of community.

Ignite a Chain of Wellness

Now that you're equipped with the insights and strategies to embrace a healthier lifestyle through fasting, it's time to share the wealth of knowledge you've gained. By sharing your honest thoughts about this book on Amazon, you're not just offering your perspective; you're guiding other women looking to transform their health and well-being to a resource that could change their lives.

Leaving a review is more than a kind gesture; it's a beacon for those searching for guidance on their journey towards improved health, hormonal balance, and vitality. Your words have the power to illuminate the path for others, helping them discover the transformative power of fasting that you've experienced.

We are deeply grateful for your support. The movement towards a healthier, more empowered life is fueled by the sharing of knowledge. By leaving your review, you're not only contributing to the growth of this community but also ensuring that the message of holistic health and fasting continues to reach and inspire more individuals.

Thank you for being a pivotal part of this journey. Together, we're not just sharing information; we're changing lives.

With heartfelt appreciation, Patricia B.

Just scan the QR code or click the link below to share your thoughts

»>Leave Amazon Review Click Here«<

Conclusion

In the concluding chapter of our journey through the transformative world of fasting, particularly for women, we've traversed a path of discovery, challenge, and triumph. This book began with a personal narrative—my struggle with postpartum weight loss, the endless cycle of diets that followed, and the serendipitous discovery of fasting as a beacon of hope and transformation. Through this lens of personal struggle and eventual enlightenment, we've explored the profound impact fasting can have on women's health, weight management, and overall well-being.

Our vision was clear from the outset: to demystify the process of fasting for women, to illuminate its potential as not just a temporary fix but a lifelong journey towards hormonal balance, weight loss, and enhanced health. This book has been meticulously crafted to serve as a comprehensive guide for women across all walks of life, aiming to seamlessly integrate fasting into their daily routines, irrespective of their age, life stage, or the complexity of their schedules.

Central to our discourse has been the recognition of women's unique physiological and hormonal landscape. We've delved into how these distinct needs shape the fasting approach, ensuring that every piece of advice and strategy is tailored to honor and address these differences. From the nuances of fasting during different phases of the menstrual cycle to the considerations required during menopause, this guide has left no stone unturned.

We've journeyed through the core principles of fasting and women's health, personalized fasting plans, advanced techniques, and the practicalities of incorporating fasting into a bustling lifestyle. Moreover, we've cast a gaze toward the horizon, contemplating the future of fasting and its evolving role in women's health.

Personalization has emerged as a cornerstone of effective fasting. We've emphasized the critical importance of tailoring fasting endeavors to align with individual health profiles, lifestyles, and the unique rhythms of women's bodies. This book has been an invitation to engage in a dynamic process of learning, experimentation, and adaptation, always with an ear to the ground, listening intently to the feedback provided by your own body.

The fasting journey is as much about community and support as it is about individual discovery. We've highlighted the invaluable role that a supportive network—virtual or physical—plays in sustaining and enriching this journey. Sharing experiences, challenges, and victories within a community bolsters individual resolve and weaves a tapestry of collective wisdom and encouragement.

Moreover, we've ventured into the mental and emotional realms of fasting, advocating for mindfulness, stress management, and nurturing a positive self-image. These facets are integral to a holistic fasting experience, reinforcing that fasting transcends mere dietary change, evolving into a profound exercise in self-care and self-awareness.

As we draw this book close, I extend a heartfelt call to action. Whether at the cusp of your fasting journey or navigating its deeper waters, I urge you to step forward with confidence and determination. Embrace fasting not merely as a dietary choice but as a lifestyle, a conscious decision towards better health and a more vibrant life.

I express my deepest gratitude to you, the reader, for embarking on this journey. Your courage to explore, adapt, and transform is the true essence of this book's spirit. When approached with care, intention, and a deep understanding of our unique needs as women, fasting holds the key to unlocking a wellspring of health and vitality.

Let this not be the end but a beginning guiding you towards continuous growth and sharing. Inspire others with your journey, teach from your experiences, and together, let us foster a culture of health, empowerment, and community among women. Here's to the transformative power of fasting, the journeys yet to be embarked upon, and the countless lives to be touched and changed.

Nutrient-Dense Food List

S pinach

- Rich in iron, magnesium, and vitamins A, C, and K.
- Supports eye health, reduces oxidative stress, and improves heart health.

Salmon

- High in omega-3 fatty acids, protein, and B vitamins.
- Benefits brain health, reduces inflammation, and lowers blood pressure.

Blueberries

- Packed with antioxidants and vitamin C.
- Promotes heart health, brain function, and anti-aging properties.

Quinoa

- Contains all nine essential amino acids, making it a complete protein source.
- High in fiber, magnesium, B vitamins, iron, potassium, calcium, phosphorus, vitamin E, and various beneficial antioxidants.

Almonds

- Rich in healthy fats, protein, magnesium, and vitamin E.
- Can lower blood sugar levels, reduce blood pressure, and lower cholesterol levels.

Avocado

- High in potassium, heart-healthy monounsaturated fats, and fiber.
- Supports heart health, reduces inflammation, and may aid in weight loss.

Sweet Potatoes

- High in beta-carotene, vitamins A and C, and fiber.
- Supports immune function, enhances brain function, and aids in eye health.

Broccoli

- Rich in vitamins C, K, and A, fiber, and antioxidants.
- Can help prevent cancer, reduce inflammation, and support heart health.

Chia Seeds

- Loaded with omega-3 fatty acids, fiber, and protein.
- Promotes digestive health, heart health, and may help in weight management.

Eggs

- High-quality protein source with vitamins D and B12.
- Supports brain health, eye health, and provides essential amino acids.

Kale

- Extremely nutrient-dense, high in vitamins A, K, C, and minerals like calcium.
- Supports bone health, has anti-inflammatory effects, and detoxifies the body.

Garlic

- Contains bioactive compounds with medicinal properties.
- Can combat sickness, improve heart health, and may have anti-cancer properties.

Walnuts

- High in omega-3 fats, antioxidants, and phytosterols.
- Supports brain health, can reduce heart disease risk, and may improve mood.

Lentils

- High in protein, fiber, and minerals like iron and potassium.
- Supports digestive health, stabilizes blood sugar, and is good for heart health.

Greek Yogurt

- Rich in probiotics, calcium, and protein.
- Supports digestive health, bone health, and can boost the immune system.

Olive Oil

- High in monounsaturated fats and antioxidants.
- Benefits heart health, has anti-inflammatory properties, and may protect against stroke.

Turmeric

- Contains curcumin, a substance with powerful anti-inflammatory and antioxidant properties.
- May improve brain function, fight chronic diseases, and reduce arthritis symptoms.

Flaxseeds

- High in omega-3 fats, fiber, and lignans.
- Can reduce cancer risk, improve cholesterol, and lower blood pressure.
- Beets
- High in fiber, folate (vitamin B9), manganese, potassium, iron, and vitamin C.
- Can improve athletic performance, help fight inflammation, and support brain health.

Pumpkin Seeds

- Packed with antioxidants, magnesium, zinc, and fatty acids.
- Supports heart health, prostate health, and protects against certain cancers.

Chicken Breast

- Lean protein source with vitamins B6 and B12.
- Supports muscle growth, bone health, and weight management.

Black Beans

- Rich in protein, fiber, and antioxidants.
- Promotes heart health, supports digestive health, and helps stabilize blood sugar.

Mushrooms

- Good source of protein, fiber, antioxidants, and B vitamins.
- Supports immune function, may have anti-cancer properties, and can promote heart health.

Apples

- High in fiber, vitamin C, and various antioxidants.
- Supports heart health, promotes digestive health, and may help manage diabetes.

Cauliflower

- Rich in vitamins C, K, and B6, fiber, and antioxidants.
- Can reduce the risk of heart disease, fight inflammation, and support hormonal balance.

Kiwi

- High in vitamin C, vitamin K, vitamin E, fiber, and potassium.
- Supports immune function, aids digestion, and can help manage blood pressure.

Cottage Cheese

- Rich in protein, B vitamins, calcium, and selenium.
- Promotes bone health, supports weight loss, and can help stabilize blood sugar levels.

Bell Peppers

- High in vitamin C, vitamin B6, and folate.

· Supports immune system, promotes eye health, and may reduce the risk of chronic diseases.

Oats

· Good source of carbs, fiber (beta-glucan), vitamins, and minerals.
· Can lower cholesterol levels, improve blood sugar control, and supports digestive health.

Tomatoes

· High in vitamin C, potassium, folate, and vitamin K.
· Supports heart health, may reduce cancer risk, and protects against sun damage.

Recipes

Chickpea and Avocado Salad

Creating a Chickpea and Avocado Salad is a simple, nutritious, and delicious way to enjoy a mix of vegetables, legumes, and healthy fats. Here's a straightforward recipe with numbered steps to guide you through the process.

Ingredients:

- 1 can (15 ounces) chickpeas, drained and rinsed
- 1 ripe avocado, peeled, pitted, and chopped
- 1/2 red onion, finely chopped
- 1/2 cucumber, chopped
- 1/2 red bell pepper, chopped
- A handful of cherry tomatoes, halved
- 1/4 cup fresh cilantro, chopped (optional)
- Juice of 1 lemon
- 2 tablespoons olive oil
- Salt and pepper, to taste
- 1 teaspoon ground cumin (optional)
- 1 clove garlic, minced (optional)

Instructions:

1. **Prepare the Ingredients**: Start by draining and rinsing the chickpeas. Peel and chop the avocado, finely chop the red onion, chop the cucumber

and red bell pepper, and halve the cherry tomatoes. If you're using cilantro, chop it as well.

2. **Make the Salad Base**: In a large mixing bowl, combine the chickpeas, avocado, red onion, cucumber, red bell pepper, and cherry tomatoes. If you're using cilantro, add it to the bowl.

3. **Dressing**: In a small bowl, whisk together the lemon juice, olive oil, minced garlic (if using), ground cumin (if using), salt, and pepper. This will be your dressing.

4. **Combine**: Pour the dressing over the salad ingredients in the large bowl. Gently toss everything together, making sure the ingredients are evenly coated with the dressing.

5. **Season**: Taste the salad and adjust the seasoning if necessary. You might want to add more salt, pepper, or lemon juice according to your preference.

6. **Serve**: The Chickpea and Avocado Salad can be served immediately or chilled in the refrigerator for about 30 minutes before serving. This allows the flavors to meld together more thoroughly.

This salad is versatile, so feel free to adjust the ingredients and their quantities based on your preferences or dietary needs. Enjoy your nutritious and flavorful Chickpea and Avocado Salad!

Quinoa and Black Bean Salad

Quinoa and Black Bean Salad is a hearty, nutritious dish that combines the health benefits of whole grains, legumes, and vegetables. This salad is packed with protein, fiber, and various vitamins and minerals, making it an excellent choice for a healthy meal. Here's how to make it, including a detailed ingredient list.

Ingredients:

- 1 cup quinoa (uncooked)
- 2 cups water
- 1 can (15 ounces) black beans, drained and rinsed

- 1 red bell pepper, chopped
- 1/4 cup fresh cilantro, chopped
- 1/4 cup red onion, finely chopped
- 1/2 cup corn (fresh, canned, or thawed from frozen)
- 1 avocado, diced
- Juice of 2 limes
- 2 tablespoons olive oil
- 1/2 teaspoon ground cumin
- Salt and pepper, to taste
- 1 clove garlic, minced (optional)
- 1 jalapeno, seeded and minced (optional for extra heat)

Instructions:

1. **Cook the Quinoa**: Rinse the quinoa under cold water in a fine mesh strainer. In a medium saucepan, bring 2 cups of water to a boil. Add the quinoa, reduce heat to low, cover, and simmer for about 15 minutes, or until the water is absorbed and the quinoa is tender. Remove from heat and let it sit covered for 5 minutes, then fluff with a fork.
2. **Prepare the Vegetables and Beans**: While the quinoa is cooking, prepare the rest of the ingredients. Drain and rinse the black beans, chop the red bell pepper, cilantro, and red onion, dice the avocado, and if using, mince the garlic and jalapeno. If you're using canned or frozen corn, make sure it's drained or thawed.
3. **Make the Dressing**: In a small bowl, whisk together the lime juice, olive oil, ground cumin, salt, and pepper. Adjust the seasoning to taste. If you're using garlic, add it to the dressing.
4. **Combine the Salad**: In a large bowl, combine the cooked quinoa, black beans, red bell pepper, cilantro, red onion, corn, and if using, jalapeno. Pour the dressing over the salad and toss until everything is well mixed.
5. **Add the Avocado**: Gently fold in the diced avocado, being careful not to mash it.
6. **Chill and Serve**: Let the salad chill in the refrigerator for at least 30

minutes before serving. This allows the flavors to meld together. Serve chilled or at room temperature.

This Quinoa and Black Bean Salad is not only delicious and easy to make but also offers a balanced combination of nutrients beneficial for overall health. Enjoy this vibrant and wholesome salad!

Salmon and Roasted Vegtables

Salmon with roasted vegetables is a wholesome, flavorful meal that's simple to prepare and packed with nutrients. This meal combines the rich, fatty texture of salmon with the earthy sweetness of roasted vegetables, making it a balanced dish that's both satisfying and healthy. Here's how to make it, including the ingredients list.

Ingredients:

- 4 salmon fillets (about 6 ounces each)
- 2 tablespoons olive oil, divided
- Salt and pepper, to taste
- 1 teaspoon dried thyme or rosemary (or a mix), divided
- 2 garlic cloves, minced
- 1 lemon, sliced into rounds
- 1 medium zucchini, cut into bite-sized pieces
- 1 red bell pepper, cut into bite-sized pieces
- 1 yellow bell pepper, cut into bite-sized pieces
- 1 small red onion, cut into wedges
- 1/2 pound small potatoes, halved or quartered (depending on size)
- Optional: fresh herbs for garnish (e.g., dill, parsley)

Instructions:

1. **Preheat the Oven**: Preheat your oven to 425°F (220°C). This high temperature is perfect for roasting vegetables and cooking salmon to perfection.

2. **Prepare the Vegetables**: In a large bowl, toss the zucchini, bell peppers, red onion, and potatoes with 1 tablespoon of olive oil, half of the minced garlic, half of the dried thyme or rosemary, and season with salt and pepper to taste. Ensure all the vegetables are evenly coated.

3. **Roast the Vegetables**: Spread the vegetables out in a single layer on a large baking sheet. Make sure they're not overcrowded to ensure they roast and don't steam. Place in the preheated oven and roast for about 20-25 minutes, or until they're tender and starting to brown. Stir once halfway through cooking.

4. **Season the Salmon**: While the vegetables are roasting, prepare the salmon. Rub the fillets with the remaining tablespoon of olive oil and season with salt, pepper, the rest of the minced garlic, and the remaining dried thyme or rosemary. Place a lemon slice on top of each fillet.

5. **Add the Salmon to the Oven**: After the vegetables have been roasting for about 15 minutes, remove the baking sheet from the oven and make space among the vegetables to place the salmon fillets. Return the baking sheet to the oven and roast for another 10-12 minutes, or until the salmon is cooked through and flakes easily with a fork.

6. **Garnish and Serve**: Once the salmon and vegetables are cooked, remove from the oven. If desired, garnish with fresh herbs like dill or parsley for added flavor and a pop of color.

7. **Enjoy**: Serve the salmon fillets alongside the roasted vegetables. This dish pairs well with a side of quinoa, rice, or a fresh salad for a complete meal.

This meal is not only delicious and easy to prepare but also offers a balanced mix of macronutrients and micronutrients, making it a great addition to a healthy diet.

Mixed Berry and Spinach Smoothie

A Mixed Berry and Spinach Smoothie is a delicious, nutrient-packed drink that combines the sweetness of berries with the health benefits of spinach. This smoothie is perfect for a quick breakfast, a post-workout snack, or a healthy afternoon pick-me-up. Here's how to make it, including the ingredients list.

Ingredients:

- 1 cup mixed berries (such as strawberries, blueberries, raspberries, and blackberries), fresh or frozen
- 1 cup fresh spinach leaves, packed
- 1 banana, peeled (for sweetness and creaminess)
- 1/2 cup Greek yogurt (for protein and a creamy texture; use plant-based yogurt for a vegan option)
- 1 cup almond milk (or any milk of your choice)
- 1 tablespoon chia seeds (optional, for added fiber and omega-3s)
- 1 tablespoon honey or maple syrup (optional, for added sweetness)
- Ice cubes (optional, if you prefer a colder smoothie or if using fresh berries)

Instructions:

1. **Prepare the Ingredients**: If you're using fresh berries, wash them thoroughly. Rinse the spinach leaves to remove any dirt or residue.
2. **Blend the Spinach and Liquid**: In a blender, combine the spinach leaves and almond milk. Blend until the mixture is smooth. Starting with the liquid helps to ensure that the spinach is fully blended and there are no leafy chunks.
3. **Add the Berries and Banana**: Add the mixed berries and banana to the blender. If you're using frozen berries, they can help chill the smoothie, so you might not need additional ice.
4. **Add Yogurt and Optional Ingredients**: Add the Greek yogurt to the blender. If you're using chia seeds for extra fiber and omega-3 fatty acids, add them now. If you prefer your smoothie a bit sweeter, add honey or maple syrup to taste.
5. **Blend Until Smooth**: Blend everything together until the mixture is smooth and creamy. If the smoothie is too thick, you can add a little

more almond milk to reach your desired consistency. If you prefer a colder smoothie and didn't use frozen berries, add a few ice cubes and blend again.

6. **Taste and Adjust**: Taste the smoothie and adjust the sweetness if necessary by adding more honey or maple syrup. If it's too thick, add a bit more milk.

7. **Serve Immediately**: Pour the smoothie into a glass or a to-go container if you're on the move. Enjoy your Mixed Berry and Spinach Smoothie right away for the best taste and texture.

This Mixed Berry and Spinach Smoothie is not only delicious but also incredibly healthy, making it a fantastic choice for anyone looking to boost their fruit and vegetable intake in a tasty way.

Kale and Sweet Potato Bowl

A Kale and Sweet Potato Bowl with roasted sweet potatoes, sautéed kale, quinoa, a fried egg, and a tahini dressing combines hearty, nutritious ingredients into a delicious and satisfying meal. This bowl is perfect for any meal of the day and offers a great balance of flavors and textures. Here's how to make it, including the ingredients list.

Ingredients:

For the Bowl:

- 2 medium sweet potatoes, peeled and diced into small cubes
- 2 tablespoons olive oil, divided
- Salt and pepper, to taste
- 1 cup quinoa, rinsed
- 2 cups water or vegetable broth
- 4 cups kale, stems removed and leaves torn into bite-sized pieces
- 4 eggs
- Optional garnishes: sliced avocado, sesame seeds, chopped nuts

For the Tahini Dressing:

- 1/4 cup tahini
- 2 tablespoons lemon juice
- 1 tablespoon maple syrup or honey
- 2-4 tablespoons warm water, as needed to thin the dressing
- Salt and pepper, to taste

Instructions:

1. **Roast the Sweet Potatoes**: Preheat your oven to 425°F (220°C). Toss the diced sweet potatoes with 1 tablespoon of olive oil and season with salt and pepper. Spread them out in a single layer on a baking sheet. Roast for about 25-30 minutes, or until tender and caramelized, stirring halfway through.

2. **Cook the Quinoa**: While the sweet potatoes are roasting, combine the rinsed quinoa and water (or vegetable broth) in a medium saucepan. Bring to a boil, then reduce heat to low, cover, and simmer for about 15 minutes, or until the liquid is absorbed. Remove from heat and let it sit covered for 5 minutes, then fluff with a fork.

3. **Sauté the Kale**: Heat 1 tablespoon of olive oil in a large skillet over medium heat. Add the kale and sauté until it is wilted and tender, about 5-7 minutes. Season with salt and pepper to taste.

4. **Fry the Eggs**: In the same skillet (or another if you prefer), fry the eggs to your liking. Season with a little salt and pepper.

5. **Prepare the Tahini Dressing**: Whisk together the tahini, lemon juice, maple syrup (or honey), and warm water until smooth. Add more water if needed to achieve a pourable consistency. Season with salt and pepper to taste.

6. **Assemble the Bowls**: Divide the quinoa among four bowls. Top each with an equal amount of the roasted sweet potatoes and sautéed kale. Place a fried egg on top of each bowl.

7. **Drizzle with Tahini Dressing**: Drizzle each bowl generously with the tahini dressing. If desired, add optional garnishes like sliced avocado, sesame seeds, or chopped nuts.

8. **Serve and Enjoy**: Your Kale and Sweet Potato Bowls are ready to serve. Enjoy this

This combination makes for a balanced meal with complex carbs, protein, healthy fats, and a wide range of vitamins and minerals, supporting overall health and well-being.

Resources

DeCesaris, L. (2023, January 18). How intermittent fasting affects women's hormones. https://www.rupahealth.com/post/how-intermittent-fasting-affects-womens-hormones

Foster, K. (2023, September 20). Intermittent fasting myths debunked: What science really says about fasting. Retrieved from https://drkimfoster.com/160-2/

Jones, J. (2023, December 6). Intermittent fasting for women: A beginner's guide. *Healthline.* https://www.healthline.com/nutrition/intermittent-fasting-for-women

Ajmera, R. (2021, March 22). Can you drink water when fasting? *Healthline.* https://www.healthline.com/nutrition/can-you-drink-water-when-fasting

Floyd, R., Gryson, R., Mockler, D., Gibney, J., Duggan, S. N., & Behan, L. A. (2022). The effect of time-restricted eating on insulin levels and insulin sensitivity in patients with polycystic ovarian syndrome: A systematic review. *PMC.* https://www.ncbi.nlm.nih.gov/pmc/articles/PMC9507776/

Nastasi, P. (2024, January 23). The best intermittent fasting apps to promote weight loss. *Sports Illustrated.* https://www.si.com/showcase/nutrition/best-intermittent-fasting-app

Brighten, J. (2023, December 29). Intermittent fasting for menopause: What you need to know before you start. Retrieved from https://drbrighten.com/intermittent-fasting-for-menopause/

Panoff, L. (2024). Menopause and intermittent fasting – Plus 5 tips for doing it right. *Midday Health*. Retrieved from https://midday.health/blog/menopause-and-intermittent-fasting-plus-5-tips-for-doing-it-rig

Roach, H. (2023, December 3). Intermittent fasting for women in menopause. *Health and Her*. https://healthandher.com/en-us/blogs/expert-advice/intermittent-fasting-menopause

Cienfuegos, S., Corapi, S., Gabel, K., Ezpeleta, M., Kalam, F., Lin, S., Pavlou, V., & Varady, K. A. (2022). Effect of intermittent fasting on reproductive hormone levels in females and males: A review of human trials. *PMC*. https://www.ncbi.nlm.nih.gov/pmc/articles/PMC9182756/

Diet Doctor. (2024). Intermittent fasting success stories: Women 40+. Retrieved from https://www.dietdoctor.com/intermittent-fasting/success-stories/women-40

Tinsley, G. (2021, April 7). What are the best foods to break a fast with? *Medical News Today*. https://www.medicalnewstoday.com/articles/what-to-eat-after-fasting

OpenAI. (2024). *ChatGPT* (4) [Large language model]. https://chat.openai.com

Levy, J. (2023, August 21). Benefits of autophagy, plus how to induce it. *Dr. Axe*. https://draxe.com/health/benefits-of-autophagy/

Zero. (2019, July 26). How to stay hydrated while fasting. *Zero Longevity*. https://zerolongevity.com/blog/how-to-stay-hydrated-while-fasting/

WebMD Editorial Contributors. (2021, October 25). Psychological benefits of fasting. *WebMD.* https://www.webmd.com/diet/psychological-benefits-of-fasting

Taubert, S. (2024). How to stop emotional eating with intermittent fasting. *BodyFast.* https://www.bodyfast.app/en/stop-emotional-eating/

Nair, P. M. K., & Khawale, P. G. (2016, April). Role of therapeutic fasting in women's health: An overview. *PMC.* https://www.ncbi.nlm.nih.gov/pmc/articles/PMC4960941/

Cole, W. (2024). Exactly how holistic women's health is helping women take back control of their health. *Dr. Will Cole.* https://drwillcole.com/functional-medicine/exactly-how-holistic-womens-health-is-helping-women-take-back-control-of-their-health

The Sport Dietitian. (2023). What is intermittent fasting? *The Sport Dietitian.* https://thesportdietitian.co.uk/is-intermittent-fasting-sustainable/

Printed in Great Britain
by Amazon

46528879R00086